Common Questions About The Liver-Cleansing Diet

1. Can I follow the diet while pregnant?

Yes you can, but only under your doctor's supervision because some pregnant women have medical conditions that may necessitate special nutritional requirements. While on the diet you should take supplements of calcium, iron, and folic acid.

2. Can I drink tea, coffee or alcohol while on the diet?

Yes you can, but restrict intake to two to three cups of tea and one cup of coffee daily. Do not drink more than three to four glasses of alcohol per week while on the diet.

3. If I want to lose weight after the eight-week menu plan can I stay on the diet?

You can stay on the diet for as long as you like, and if weight loss is slow or comes to a plateau, eat smaller meals.

4. Can I follow the diet if I am a diabetic?

Yes you can, but stay with your doctor's supervision, and remember to have regular snacks using foods from our menus to prevent hypoglycemia.

5. Do I need to take nutritional supplements while on the diet?

If you are female it is a good idea to take supplements of calcium and iron, as it is a dairy-free diet.

6. Once I finish the eight-week menu plan of the liver-cleansing diet can I eat red meat?

If you like red meat you may eat it, provided it is fresh and lean. Restrict red meat to two to three times weekly.

7. Will the liver-cleansing diet help me if I have liver disease?

Yes, the liver-cleansing diet will help those with liver diseases such as fatty liver, hepatitis, cirrhosis, and gall bladder disease.

8. Does this book only apply to people who want to lose weight?

No, the liver-cleansing diet will not result in weight loss, unless you are overweight, as it balances your metabolism. Many sick people are underweight and by improving their liver function will increase their appetite and maintain or gain weight. By improving liver function the load upon the immune system is reduced and many illnesses caused by inflammation or chronic infections will be gradually overcome.

If we haven't answered your question and you need further information, please write to Dr. Cabot at the Women's Health Advisory Network, 13910 North Frank Lloyd Wright Blvd., Suite 2A–101, Scottsdale, AZ. 85260 **or visit us on the internet at www.whas.com.au**

A WORD FROM DR CABOT

Dear Reader,

As an author it is very gratifying to receive positive feedback from readers about one's work. Since *The Liver-Cleansing Diet* book was released in June 1996, I have received thousands of testimonials as to the healing effects of this diet for people with diverse health problems and diseases, which further vindicates my discovery that one can cure many diseases simply by cleansing the liver. One cannot be healthy without a healthy liver and yet most people never give the liver a second thought.

If you are battling with poor health and getting nowhere I urge you to start thinking about your liver. This is so vital that in many cases it can not only cure and prevent common chronic illnesses, it really could save your life. I do not say this lightly as I am a scientific doctor who has been practicing medicine for over twenty five years and I have often been faced with difficult challenges. I have great faith in the Liver-Cleansing Diet as I have seen it work many miracles where all else has failed.

The Liver-Cleansing Diet is not a trendy weight loss diet (although it is extremely effective for obesity). In contrast, it will become established as a household name for a long, long time because people who have used it sing its praises far and wide. Many fad diets come and go and indeed may be dangerous or make you miserable because they are far too restrictive and difficult to follow. In contrast, the Liver-Cleansing Diet is easy and safe and is really a form of awareness or consciousness which will give you the key to a strong immune system and healthy blood vessels.

Furthermore, the Liver-Cleansing Diet is **not** a "kill joy" diet which only goodie goodies can follow. After the eight-week cleansing, you may continue to enjoy nice wines and spirits and, if you desire, lean fresh red meats in moderation. If you don't want to follow the eight-week plan, then that's OK too, simply follow the twelve vital principles for a healthy liver (see chapter 5) and pick and choose recipes and foods that you enjoy.

Since this book became a best seller I have had a small number of critics (only two so far) from the medical profession and this has taught me a lot. One of these critics said that my diet was "anti-science" and encouraged people to stay away from their doctors. In the front of this book I state categorically that patients should remain with their own doctors and that this book is not a substitute for your doctor's care. Please always have your regular check ups and talk to your doctor. I have a very close friend who now has advanced cancer which was not diagnosed simply because she didn't go to a doctor for twenty years. I am not "alternative" as this is a meaningless term but rather I am proud to state that my book is practical commonsense science.

See for yourself—the proof of the pudding is in the eating!

My other critic stated that my book is no more than a "low-fat cook book" which really amazed me and showed me just how little many so-called "liver experts" know about nutrition. The Liver-Cleansing Diet is

not a low-fat diet, but rather contains plenty of the correct types of fats (natural fatty acids) for healthy liver function. The most amazing thing of all is that these two critics bagged my book without first talking to me about my results or case histories and neither of them had tried the diet on any of their sick patients to see if it really worked! How can anyone know the benefits of a particular diet or therapy without evaluating its effects upon patients first!

So, luckily, I have a sense of humor and a belief in my results and the power of nutritional medicine or I may have been "put in my place"! Thankfully, we live in a democracy and have freedom of thought and speech although some would wish it otherwise. I would also like to ask, do these critics have all the answers for the thousands of patients who suffer with overburdened immune systems, chronic fatigue, obesity, fatty livers, and recurring blocked arteries—even after bypass surgery? Let's not suffer from what I call the "fossilized brain syndrome" where lateral and original thinking becomes a crime.

Remember that a healthy liver will reduce depression and moodiness enabling you to laugh more and not get too overheated or as the Chinese say "gung ho" about life's little tribulations.

I have chosen a small collection of genuine testimonials (names have been changed) to give you inspiration and motivation to "Love your Liver and Live Longer".

May God bless your liver and give you good health,
Yours sincerely,
Dr Sandra Cabot

TESTIMONIALS

Dear Dr Cabot,
When I saw you on the "Midday Show", I thought hoorah, as you were talking about all of my problems and offered hope. I told my friend and we rushed out to buy your book, even though we did not think it would help us that much as we are in our late 60s.

Your liver diet has helped me clear up some long-term personal problems that were really getting me down.

I no longer wake up at night with hot sweats.
The bloated feeling I always had has gone.
My indigestion has gone and I no longer need antacids.
The black circles under my eyes have gone.
I have lost 13 pounds in eight weeks.
The most important one is that my blood pressure is now normal.

My doctor says that if it stays down I will no longer need any medication. This is after many years of suffering with high blood pressure.

So all I can say is a big THANK YOU and thanks to the Women's Health Advisory Service for all their help on the phone.

I am yours, a lot lighter and fitter,

Mrs K., NSW, Australia

Dear Dr Cabot,

Thank you for your wonderful eating plan. My husband, my mother, and I all went on the Liver-Cleansing Diet and we have each lost around 14 pounds. The most amazing thing happened to my baby while I was on your plan. I know the Liver Diet was not designed for breast-feeding women, however, when I read your book I felt it was not going to mean any drastic changes but more so cutting out rubbish and snack food. My son (now 14 months old) has had eczema from 5 months of age. I took him to an iridologist; (someone who examines the iris for signs of disease), who said his eyes were too dark and that his liver was not functioning properly. After 4 weeks on your program I returned to the iridologist at the health food store and asked him to have another look at my son's eyes. After looking, he was very surprised and said that his eyes were a clear deep brown color with the various pigments clearly visible. He was suitably impressed and said there was significant improvement. Knowing that I was still breast feeding he asked what I was doing differently. I pointed to your book on the counter and he smiled and said "That does not surprise me, it's a wonderful diet". So what I find interesting is the possibilities for nursing mothers and benefits for their babies.

I tried different eating plans but my weight didn't shift until the liver cleanser. I feel great, my baby is healthy and happy and my husband is getting lots of compliments on how much healthier and slimmer he looks. Mom has been on every diet put to paper and she has never found one she really likes—until now. She looks the best she's looked in a long time. Thank you Sandra.

From Mrs H, Victoria, Australia

Here's an interesting case history for animal lovers!

Dear Dr Cabot,

Kala Beat was named the 1995 "Horse of the Year" in the Northern Rivers Racing Association area (Australia). The last 2 times that he raced the trainer R.G. Gosling noticed the horse was not finishing his races and ordered a blood count to check for problems. The veterinarian found that the horse's liver enzyme count was too high with a reading of 90. The normal liver reading for a horse is up to 30. The horse always had a liver reading higher than normal but it had never escalated to 90. We heard about the liver tonic powder called "Livatone" and the great results with humans taking this product. So it was decided we would give Kala Beat a treatment using the Livatone. After checking, we were told that the horse would need 4 times the usual human dose. We also increased the carrots and sunflower seeds in his diet. After being on this treatment for a month another blood count was taken and the liver count had dropped from 90 to 37. This was a better liver count than our horse had ever had. After 6 weeks another blood count was taken and the liver count is now down to 33.

Regards,
Lyn Gosling
Let's hope that Kala Beat starts winning again!

Good morning Dr Cabot! (sent by fax)
This is to advise you of the most wonderful result which I have had from the Liver-Cleansing Diet. I saw you in April and after a blood test my liver result was really bad to say the least. I am not a drinker, if you can call maybe 2 glasses of wine a week drinking. I am 54 years old and have never had more than 2 drinks even at a party as my system feels its effects immediately. In September I had to have all sorts of tests, including a blood test, to purchase insurance. Guess what—not a slight problem showed up with the liver!!!! Completely normal!!!! I started on the liver tonic powder in juices (beet, carrot, celery and apple) twice a day, although this was interrupted during my travels in the USA. I also gave up dairy products and lost 10 pounds easily.

Your book contains more answers than I have ever had, my health has improved and for the first time ever I have lost weight.
Congratulations and heartfelt thanks,
Ms F., Sydney, Australia

Dear Dr Cabot,
I am taking this opportunity to write to you and tell you of the effect your liver-cleansing diet had on me. For several years I have had a slowly worsening health problem which has caused many and varied symptoms, ranging from allergic problems to finally, late in 1995, a diagnosis by a hepatologist of sclerosing cholangitis. I was told that there was no specific treatment for this condition apart from more exercise, eat less, etc., and that there was no known cure for the condition at present. For the last 12 months or so I followed this advice and can honestly say that apart from the symptoms getting worse, deep itching, and a general yellow color, along with a feeling of being unwell at all times, nothing changed. It was in early August that I came across

your book. I started the diet at the beginning of September and followed carefully your 8-week plan. The day after finishing your diet I had a liver function test done by my local doctor and have since seen the specialist and the results are nothing less than amazing.

Gamma enzyme down from 256 to 52.

Cholesterol down from 220 to 120 mg/dl

Weight loss of 28 pounds over the 8 weeks.

This is only 3 items and I cannot quote the others but overall everything had dramatically decreased and both doctors were nothing short of amazed with the results. Of course, they had little comment on your book but both had the same advice of "whatever you are doing, keep doing it". Doctor, while a few of your colleagues seem to be loathe to comment on your book's success, please accept my personal thanks for a job well done. I can assure you that after the results I have had many of our friends are now on the diet and hoping for a similar outcome. As well, while I was on your diet my wife also lost well over 14 pounds for the 2 months and we have decided to stick to the diet in parts for the future.

Regards and most sincere thanks,

Mr R.H., Newcastle, NSW, Australia

Dear Dr Cabot, (here's one e-mailed from the internet)

I am writing on behalf of a friend in the USA. I have used your LCD with great success. I had high cholesterol and triglyceride levels and am Hep C positive. I followed your diet and feel a lot better for it. Cholesterol and triglyceride levels are back to normal, liver count is normal and I can now fit back into 7 pairs of Levi's that I'd put out of commission. I have suggested your book on the "Hepatitis News Group" as a source of hope for those suffering from active Hepatitis C.

From Ms M., newsgroup internet

Dear Dr Cabot,

I am writing to let you know that I tried your LCD for 8 weeks and I have not felt this good for a long time. Four years ago I discovered that I had Hep C and my liver tests have never been normal in all that time. Just before starting the LCD my ALT liver enzymes were 158. After 3 weeks they were 127 and at the end of your 8-week program they were 57. My doctor said all the other tests were normal.

I was also taking Livatone and Echinacea. I was due to see a hepatologist yesterday, but on learning that my tests were normal, a sister at St Vincent's Hospital advised me not to go in. She also has Hep C and was just starting your LCD. She asked me if I would write to the hospital and tell them my results as they don't believe in it or herbal

medicines. I have now changed my way of eating and can only hope that I stay feeling this healthy. It is wonderful not to feel tired all the time.
Yours sincerely,
Ms B, Melbourne, Vic

Fax sent to one of the two colleagues who have criticized the diet.
Dear Doctor (name undisclosed),
Having watched "A Current Affair" on TV, I would like to tell you of my experience. I am a registered nurse and am still practicing. During the past few years I have not enjoyed good health but since following Dr Cabot's diet my lifestyle has taken a complete turn around. Not only have I lost 28 pounds, I no longer suffer with diabetes (previously controlled with medication). I no longer require HRT which I had used for 25 years following a hysterectomy at age 26.

I have endless energy and my general well-being is excellent. It's a pity that some "high flying medicos" do not take a more holistic approach when assessing patients. In my field of work the trend is changing towards holistic medicine with great success. If patients could receive the holistic treatment they deserve we could save the country millions of dollars.
Ms W., Registered nurse, Sydney, Australia

Dear Dr Cabot,
I have just completed the LCD and have lost 22 pounds. The LCD has changed my eating habits dramatically. Understanding how the liver works and experiencing the symptoms of "fatty liver" has made me realize what I have been doing to my body over many years. I am 47 years old, 5 foot 3 inches, and weighed 200 pounds. I had a problem losing weight even though I did not eat excessively. Indeed, the less I ate the more I would put on, and then, disappointed I had not lost any weight, I would eat the wrong foods and rapidly gain weight.

Your LCD is so different from regular diets I have tried because it is the first diet to remove the fat from my liver so that my liver can start burning fat for the first time in many years. Before reading your book I had no idea that the liver was the major fat burning organ in the body. Thank you for the book and my healthy liver.
Ms K, South Australia

Dear Dr Cabot,
I have been following your LCD for 4 weeks and I feel marvelous. I have lost 9 pounds in weight and can fit into some of my nice clothes again. I am in my early forties and was starting to notice little unexplained aches

and pains that I put down to "getting older", but in the last 4 weeks these aches and pains have either disappeared or are hardly noticeable. To add to my joy in discovering this lifestyle my tired looking skin again has a "glow" about it which even my friends have commented upon. Thank you for putting your time into researching the effects the liver has on the body.
With thanks,
Ms H, ACT, Australia

Verbal statement from a gentleman at my seminar in Canberra, Australia, September 1996
Dr Cabot, I am here tonight to tell you and the audience that your theories on the liver are correct. Four months ago I had a severe auto-immune disease and vasculitis and was very overweight. I was dependent upon immuno-suppressant drugs and was seriously ill. Over the last four months I have been following your LCD and I have achieved great success. I have lost several pounds in weight and no longer need any of these drugs. Furthermore my diseases have completely gone. I can highly recommend your diet to everyone here tonight.

Dear Dr Cabot,
I am writing to tell you that your diet has helped my facial skin rash diagnosed as "acne rosacea". This started to break out as a pimply red burning rash upon my cheeks 10 months ago at which time I went to a doctor and was given a prescription for a tetracycline antibiotic. I took this for nearly 6 months and unfortunately it damaged my liver and caused a photosensitivity rash on my face so that it turned a bright purple-red color. In horror I rushed back to the doctor and was told to stop the antibiotics and take cortisone to suppress the purple rash. This worked but unfortunately caused severe heart palpitations (atrial fibrillation). So I stopped everything and the acne rosacea returned with a vengeance. Then I saw a naturopath who told me that skin rashes and acne rosacea are a sign of an unhealthy liver and I was advised to start your LCD. I also took some antioxidant vitamins, selenium (selemite B), and evening primrose oil. After following your LCD for 11 weeks my acne rosacea has gone completely and I have lost over 48 pounds in weight which is wonderful. Thank you for showing me that the liver has such an important effect upon the immune system.
Yours sincerely,
Ms J., Sydney, Australia

The
LIVER-
Cleansing
Diet

Sandra Cabot M.D., is a well-known media doctor and author of the best selling books: *Women's Health, Don't Let Your Hormones Ruin Your Life, The Body Shaping Diet, Menopause—HRT and its Natural Alternatives, Boost Your Energy* and *The Healthy Liver and Bowel Book.*

Sandra is a consultant to the Australian Women's Health Advisory Service, has regularly appeared in many national TV shows, has her own talk-back radio show, writes for a national women's magazine's and is a much sought after public speaker on nutritional medicine, hormonal disorders, and naturopathic medicine.

Sandra is sometimes known as the "flying doctor" as she frequently flies herself to many of Australia's country towns to hold health forums for rural women. These help to raise funds for local women's health services. She spent considerable time working in the Department of Obstetrics and Gynecology in a large missionary hospital in the Himalayan foothills of India.

With the publication of *The Liver-Cleansing Diet* in the United States of America, Sandra is at last able to share her significant experience and knowledge with men and women all over America.

Dr Sandra Cabot's books are available in America from book stores, and from SCB by calling 623 334 3232.

The
LIVER-
Cleansing
Diet

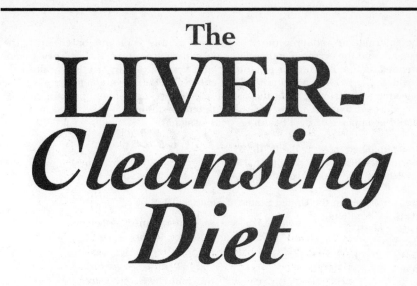

USA Edition

Sandra Cabot MD

This book will be a revelation to those
who suffer from poor health, liver
disease, and excessive weight.
I have dedicated it to all those people.

SCB International Inc.

First published in Australia in 1996
Reprinted 1996, 1997 (six times), 1999 (two times), 2000 (two times)
4th Edition Dec 2000 (two times), 2001

First published in the United States of America 1997 by
S.C.B. International
PO Box 5070
Glendale AZ
85312 - 5070
Phone 623 334 3232

Internet address: www.doctorcabot.com or
liverdoctor.com

ISBN 0 646 27789 8

Our delightful cartoons were drawn by
the talented artist Karen Barbouttis

CONTENTS

Chapter 1

INTRODUCTION TO THE LIVER-CLEANSING DIET

Many people struggle with excessive weight and sluggish metabolism all their lives and find that as they age they gradually gain more weight and become resigned to a large protruding abdomen and stubborn fat deposits. After years of going from one fad diet to the next which leads them on a "yo-yo" journey to ever increasing weight and frustration they become resigned to the misconception that nothing can ever possibly lead to lasting relief for them. There is obviously something wrong, a missing key or link, and yet although we have computers, the internet, sophisticated global satellite navigation systems, babies for postmenopausal women, and other mind boggling achievements, it seems even more mind boggling that someone has not said, "Hey, why do we have all these overweight, unhappy and unhealthy people who cannot find a solution?" In life, real solutions are generally simple (not simplistic) and they are logical and practical. They must also be easy to follow, otherwise we will fall by the wayside and they are thrown into the too hard basket!

I must admit it took me more than twenty years of medical practice before the solution dawned on me! The liver, the supreme organ of metabolism had to be the missing key. It seemed so simple and yet so incredible; why hadn't someone thought of this before?

Because with modern-day medicine we have become side-tracked into treating the symptoms of disease and not the causes. Excessive weight is a symptom of liver dysfunction and not solely due to the number of calories you eat. We have been attacking the symptom of weight excess with fad diets, obsessional high-impact aerobic exercise, stomach stapling, and toxic drugs such as appetite

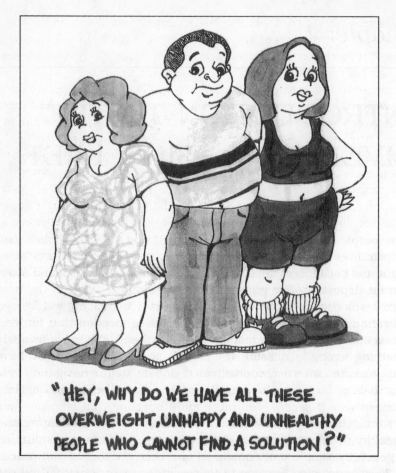

"HEY, WHY DO WE HAVE ALL THESE OVERWEIGHT, UNHAPPY AND UNHEALTHY PEOPLE WHO CANNOT FIND A SOLUTION?"

suppressants, laxatives, and diuretics. We have failed to treat the underlying cause of liver dysfunction and indeed we have managed to virtually ignore the hardest working organ in the body, with dire consequences. As you will discover in this book the consequences of mistreating the liver are not only obesity, but a higher incidence of cardiovascular and degenerative diseases that are the scourge of modern-day affluent societies.

I have seen more than 30,000 patients, many of whom have struggled with excess weight and sluggish metabolism and yet it was not until 1994 that I decided to treat all these cases with a program to improve liver function. This strategy seemed so obvious that I could have kicked myself for taking so long and yet I also felt a great sense of relief as I knew that from now on my work would be much easier and more productive. I felt a sense of urgency to bring relief to my patients and to document my new discovery. This I have been doing for two years and my theory that the liver holds the key to weight control has been vindicated in all the 1540 patients that I have treated with my program to improve liver function. The success rate, as measured by parameters of weight loss and general well-being has been 100 per cent in the patients I have been able to see regularly for monitoring. The others who live too far away to follow up myself are being monitored by correspondence and provided they continue to apply my principles for the Liver-Cleansing Diet and program they should be able to match the results I am getting with my regular patients. I have included some of the more interesting case histories of these success stories for you in this book as this will inspire and motivate you.

No matter how bad you feel your weight problem is or what you have tried before, this special Liver-Cleansing Diet can work for you. I know this to be true as I have seen it work in extremely difficult patients, some of whom had really given up hope.

I had studied the liver as a medical student and hospital intern, although in this context most of the liver patients I cared for had serious diseases of the liver, such as cirrhosis, chronic hepatitis, liver cancer or tumors, fatty livers, or liver failure—not a pretty sight. I felt much compassion for these patients as they felt terrible and their futures were in doubt, that is without the life saving surgery of liver transplant.

As a medical student I spent many hours sitting in with leading naturopathic doctors as I was intrigued by their natural healing techniques. I believed they had much to teach me and their patient waiting lists were always very long with cases that other doctors had not been able to help. It was with such naturopaths that I first learned of the tremendous importance of the largest organ in the body—the LIVER! The adult liver weighs about 42 to 53 ounces (2 pounds 10 ounces to 3 pounds 5 ounces) and comprises one fiftieth of the total adult body weight. Yes, it takes up a lot of space and is not simply there for extra padding! In all their patients naturopathic doctors examine the state of the liver through various techniques such as iridology, acupuncture pulse techniques and from the patient's history. In the vast majority of cases a liver problem would be found, sometimes only of subtle degree, sometimes quite gross, and correction of this poor liver state was always a vital step in their healing program. They would treat the liver with dietary changes and specific liver herbs and in more toxic cases with fasting programs.

I did see many positive therapeutic results, and indeed some miraculous results in very ill patients, from such treatments and came to understand that to restore good health one must ALWAYS consider the state of the liver. However, subsequently my career led me into obstetrics, gynecology, and gynecological endocrinology and the importance of considering the liver in every patient gradually slipped into my subconscious mind. Thankfully, one day I would remember to take a leaf out of the book of this old naturopathic wisdom.

I breathed a great sigh of relief, and so did my patients, when I

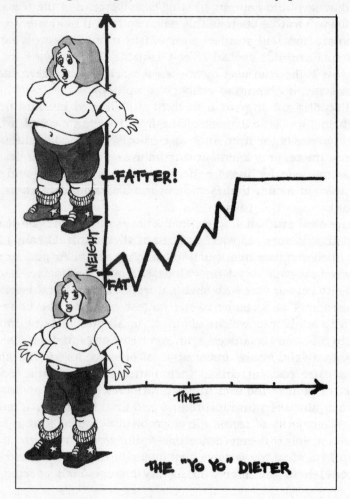

THE "YO YO" DIETER

realized the need to treat the liver with the supreme importance it deserves. I see many difficult cases where people have been chronically ill or obese for years, and they often come to see me saying that "you are my last hope" or "you are my last resort". This is a big responsibility and sometimes I think life would be much easier if they came to see me just for a sore throat; but then again medicine would not be so interesting! I feel very confident that I can help these people now that I am using a liver-cleansing and healing program. It is quite amazing how these patients can feel my confidence and enthusiasm for this type of treatment and they are all fascinated to learn how the liver holds the key to weight loss and balanced metabolism. Indeed they love this concept as it gives them an explanation as to why all those "yo yo" diets have failed and why the drugs they are taking to control problems such as blood pressure, high cholesterol, allergies etc., are not as effective as they would hope.

There are millions of women and men currently struggling with a new crash diet, spending hundreds of dollars in weight loss clinics, frantically going to the gym, and generally feeling deprived and miserable. Sure it's vital to exercise and obtain some psychological support and I believe that support groups such as Weight Watchers and Overeaters Anonymous and many others are most beneficial. But you know that you should be getting better results for the huge amount of effort you are putting in and don't know how long you can keep this hard work going. I don't blame you, it's just too hard!

You can now breathe a sigh of relief and relax about all of this, because you too have discovered the liver, which will hold the key to efficient metabolism, weight control, and good general health for you.

The liver is the major fat-burning organ in the body. If you follow the Liver-Cleansing Diet your metabolism will improve in leaps and bounds and you will start to burn fat! Conversely, if you eat the wrong foods your liver will actually make more fat so that you keep on storing fat. To a large degree, its not how much you eat, its what you eat that's far more important. When you follow the Liver-Cleansing Diet you eat delicious liver-cleansing and liver-friendly foods and your liver will then give a big sigh of relief and merrily get on with its job of regulating metabolism and burning fat. Then the process of weight loss begins naturally and without excessive effort on your part. In the Liver-Cleansing Diet you do not have to count calories or pedantically weigh every morsel of food and even better you never have to go hungry. Simply stick to the foods in the Liver-

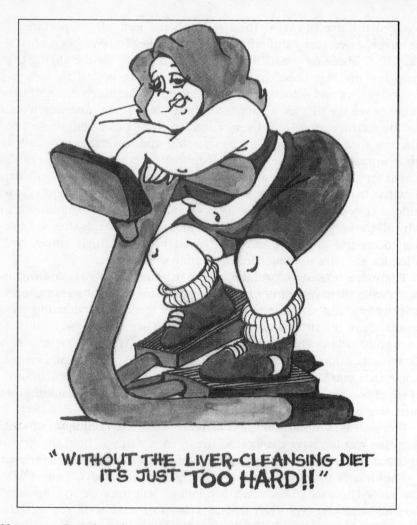

" WITHOUT THE LIVER-CLEANSING DIET
ITS JUST *TOO HARD!!* "

Cleansing Diet (LCD) and if you feel hungry eat more of these types of foods until you are satisfied.

There are twelve VITAL PRINCIPLES you need to follow to improve your liver function and these are discussed on pages 45 to 65. You will obtain even better results if you follow the eight-week menu plan of the Liver-Cleansing Diet and this is all laid out in an easy-to-follow plan on pages 81 to 105. To enhance this program I have included natural therapies for liver-cleansing and healing on pages 66 to 71.

Chapter 2

WHO CAN BENEFIT FROM THE LCD?

Everyone can benefit from the Liver-Cleansing Diet as it is designed to improve overall health and immune function. Those who are in greatest need of this diet are persons with the following health complaints.

1. EXCESSIVE BODY WEIGHT

The most accurate way of determining just how overweight you are is a ratio called the Body Mass Index (BMI). The BMI is worked out by dividing your weight by your height squared (height multiplied by height).

Body Mass Index (BMI) is a scientific way of determining how overweight you are.

$$BMI = \frac{WEIGHT\ (KILOGRAMS)}{HEIGHT \times HEIGHT\ (METERS)}$$

For example if you weigh 75 kilograms and are 1.69 meters (169 centimeters) tall then your

$$BMI = \frac{75\ kilograms}{1.69 \times 1.69\ meters}$$

$$= \frac{75}{2.856}$$

$$= 26.26\ \text{(use an electronic calculator)}$$

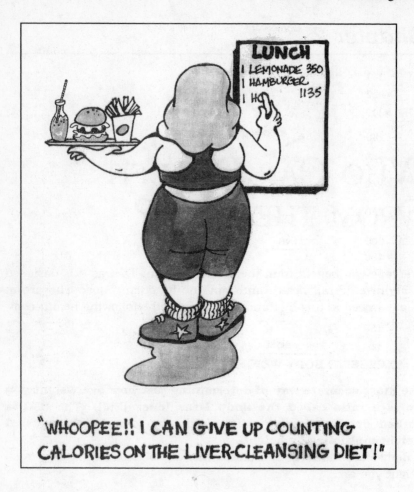

"WHOOPEE!! I CAN GIVE UP COUNTING CALORIES ON THE LIVER-CLEANSING DIET!"

If you don't like equations you can easily work out your BMI from the scale on page 15. To use it, place a ruler between your weight (undressed) and your height (without shoes). Then read your BMI ON THE MIDDLE SCALE.

If you are female you should aim to keep your BMI between 19 and 25 depending upon your build (higher values are found within this range for those with large and heavy bones). For males BMI should fall in the range of 20 to 26.

Overweight is considered between the upper limit of normal BMI (25 for women and 26 for men) and a BMI of 29. Obesity is defined as a BMI greater than 29.

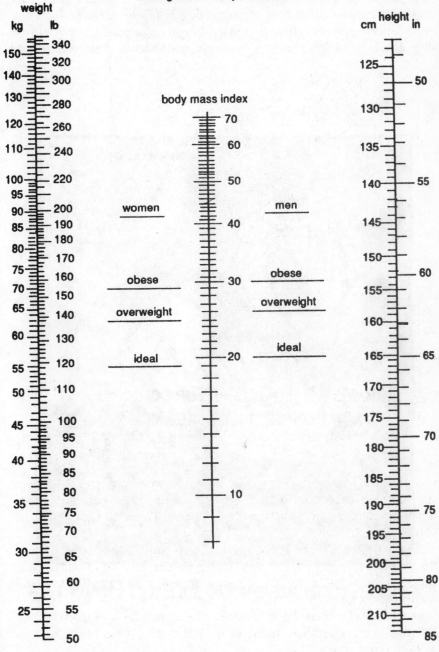

Nomogram for body mass index

If you keep your BMI within the normal range you will reduce your risk of cardiovascular disease, many degenerative diseases, diabetes, and cancer, and will enjoy increased longevity and a higher quality of life. The LCD makes this easy because any time you find your weight

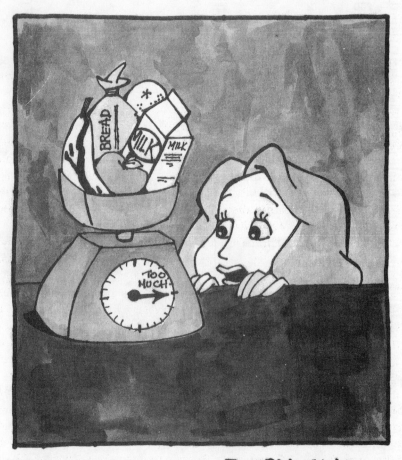

" GOODBYE TO WEIGHING EVERYTHING I EAT "

creeping up above the upper limit of BMI you can just return to the delicious menus in this book and your liver function will improve. After a few weeks weight loss will occur automatically as fat metabolism becomes more efficient. There will be no need to painstakingly weigh foods or count calories as the aim of the LCD is not to restrict your food intake. Rather, we want to merely divert you away from liver-toxic foods to liver-cleansing foods so that your liver can recommence its work of fat metabolizer.

2. LIVER DISEASE

Liver disease can take many forms and have many causes and some people have liver disease for which the medical profession can never find a cause—this is called idiopathic.

The most common causes of liver disease are alcohol excess, viral hepatitis (viruses A, B, C and others), drug abuse (especially intravenous), adverse reactions to various pharmaceutical drugs (such as analgesics, anti-inflammatory drugs, some antibiotics and antifungal drugs, and immuno-suppressants). The causes of liver disease are too numerous to mention; however, I have seen liver disease result from auto-immune diseases such as Lupus and many infections such as HIV (AIDS), malaria and tuberculosis.

Liver disease can result from exposure to occupational and environmental toxins such as insecticides, pesticides, and organic solvents. Many aromatic and chlorinated solvents are carcinogenic. They build up in the fatty areas of the body including the liver and brain. Certain occupations expose you to a higher concentration of liver toxic chemicals. Such occupations are shoe manufacturers, pest controllers, insecticide users, workers in the plastic and rubber industries, furniture and cabinet makers, hair dressers, dry cleaners, and painters.

The liver is a common site of cancer and many primary cancers from other body organs eventually spread to the liver where they grow, destroying the surrounding liver tissue. The liver is also a common site for a cancer to start, which is logical as it bears the brunt of all the toxic foods and chemicals that we ingest over a lifetime. I have also seen a case of polycystic liver in which the liver was so grossly enlarged with huge cysts that it filled the entire abdomen. Polycystic liver disease is a genetic defect that is inherited although it is not common.

Many liver diseases are short lived or acute and this is because the liver has remarkable powers of self repair and regeneration and a complete recovery usually occurs. However, if the liver is severely damaged or the noxious influence attacking it is sustained or chronic, such as in some cases of viral B and C hepatitis or persistent alcohol excess, then the liver has less likelihood of complete recovery. After many years of chronic liver inflammation and toxicity the liver can become severely scarred and distorted—this is called cirrhosis.

A relatively common cause of unexplained (idiopathic) liver disease seen in affluent societies today is a diet high in saturated and damaged fats and refined sugars. After many years on such a diet the condition of "fatty liver" may occur where the liver is swollen with fatty deposits. Fatty liver is a degenerative disease of the liver where the liver cells are literally choked to death by globules of fatty substances within them. These patients have a total inability to metabolize fats and suffer with weight excess.

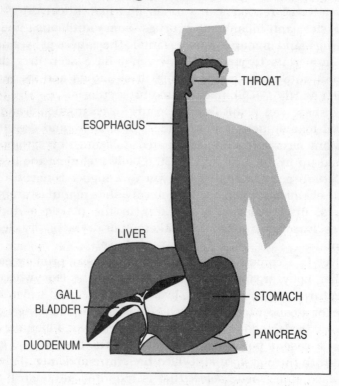

The upper digestive tract.

TESTS FOR LIVER DISEASE

If you suspect that your liver is not working properly or may be diseased ask your doctor to check your liver. The liver can be seen with various imaging techniques, such as ultrasound scanning or CAT scanning, which are done by a radiologist. An ultrasound scan of the upper abdomen will show the size and shape of the liver, gallbladder, spleen, and pancreas. CAT scanning is used to check for cancer or tumors of the liver.

Blood tests can check levels of serum bilirubin and bile acids, which may be elevated in certain types of liver and gallbladder disease. If the bilirubin is too high you may also notice that your bowel actions are very pale and that your urine is a darker color because bilirubin is diverted from the bowels to the urine.

Blood tests to measure the levels of the liver enzymes may show abnormally high levels if the liver cells are damaged or ruptured, causing them to release their intracellular enzymes into the blood stream. The liver enzymes that are measured are called alkaline phosphatase (ALK.PHOS), gamma glutamyl transpeptidase (gamma-GT), glutamic oxaloacetic transaminase (SGOT), and glutamic pyruvic transaminase (SGPT).

In the early stages of liver disease where there is only minimal damage to the liver cells there is often only a very slight elevation of the liver transaminase enzymes (SGOT and SGPT) in the blood test.

In those who consume excessive alcohol a common finding in the blood test is an elevation of the liver enzyme gamma-GT. This is often an isolated finding and the other liver enzymes are usually normal, at least in mild cases of liver damage from alcohol excess.

In patients with chronic liver diseases and in some with gallbladder disease there is a large increase in the levels of the blood fats, total cholesterol, and triglycerides. This is to be expected because the liver is the major organ for overall fat balance and metabolism. Some of these patients develop a fatty liver and may also have yellow fatty lumps growing in the skin around the eyes and on the limbs. These subcutaneous lumps of fat are called xanthomas and if these are starting to grow under your skin, they are probably accumulating in other parts of your body such as your liver, heart, kidneys, pancreas, lymph nodes, and arteries (atherosclerosis). These diseases of fatty degeneration are choking your vital organs and blood vessels and are due to the inability of your liver to metabolize the excessive and damaged fats that you have been feeding it for too long. Thankfully the

LCD can reverse this process as it will restore the ability of your obese liver to burn fat efficiently once again. Those with a fatty liver and/or high blood fats should also take a liver tonic containing taurine and lecithin (see page 66), to improve liver function.

Other tests can be done to check the ability of the liver to manufacture its vital proteins. These are tests for the proteins albumin, prothrombin, and various globulins and they show characteristic abnormalities in those whose liver function is abnormal.

This may sound rather technical, however your doctor can easily do all these tests from two or three small vials of collected blood.

In the early stages of liver disease there may be no dramatic symptoms and thus you and your doctor may be totally unaware that there is an underlying problem. Often the early stages of liver disease are found coincidentally on a routine blood test that includes tests for liver function. Chronic liver disease passes through a long period of minimal vague symptoms until the final stages of jaundice and mental confusion appear.

In my medical practice where I do a lot of routine blood tests for hormone levels and liver function in overweight patients, I often find slight elevations in liver enzymes which signifies mild impairment of liver function and slight liver damage. This can easily be reversed with the LCD and specific liver tonics as discussed on page 66. I have found that it is very difficult for many of my overweight patients to lose weight even though they may be eating only normal amounts, unless I first improve their liver function. Once they are five to six weeks into the LCD their liver-function tests are usually back to normal and the process of weight loss takes on increased momentum. Yes, the liver is the strategic organ for those who have found it very difficult to lose weight or simply just to maintain a healthy weight as they get older.

3. GALLBLADDER DISEASE

If you have gallstones (either new or recurrent gallstones) you should definitely follow the LCD as this way of eating will correct the chemical imbalance in your bile that is leading to gallstones. In many cases of gallstones it is possible to dissolve them provided you can stick with the LCD in the long term. In those who have had their gallbladder removed it is still important to follow the LCD and the twelve vital principles to improve liver function found on pages 45 to 65. This is logical if you think about it, as it was the poor quality of bile that was made by an overburdened liver on a high-fat diet that led to the gall-stones. This imbalance will remain if you don't eat liver-friendly foods and even though the gallbladder has been removed, problems often crop up again in a nearby area causing such things as pancreatitis, biliary tract disease, or fatty liver. I have found that many patients gain weight after removal of the gallbladder because their liver function remains suboptimal.

OTHER HEALTH PROBLEMS HELPED BY THE LCD

When I first designed the LCD several years ago with the aim of helping those with stubborn weight problems or liver disease, I did not realize that I would observe its powerful healing and balancing effects in many other seemingly unrelated health problems. On many occasions I have been amazed to watch this diet, over a period of four to twelve weeks, overcome problems that in the past I may have felt obligated in the first instance to treat with drugs. In many patients drugs can be avoided through the use of this diet, although in some acute problems drug therapy will be necessary and the LCD can be used simultaneously.

Let me recount to you such a case history; the details are factual but the patient's name has been changed. Christine, a 40-year-old, came to see me because she wanted to lose weight (she weighed 89 kilograms = 14 stone = 196 pounds, and was 167.5 cms = 67 inches tall, putting her BMI at 31.72.) and she also felt depressed and exhausted although she did not have an unduly stressful life. She was alarmed when I told her that her blood pressure was moderately elevated at 175/100 and that her liver was slightly unhappy with minimal elevation of liver enzymes and high cholesterol. She said to me that she could expect her mother to have these problems, but not herself, as she still considered herself young. Her diet was typical of someone with these problems—she loved cheeses, margarine, butter, salty foods, and the occasional takeout with the kids. She had two to four pieces of fruit per week and 90 per cent of her vegetables were cooked. I started Christine on the Liver-Cleansing Diet and ordered some tests to see why her blood pressure was up. I said that if her blood pressure remained high I would probably need to start her on anti-hypertensive medication. I did not realize that I had shocked her so much. When she returned eight weeks later she told me that she had left our first visit feeling like an old woman with multiple ail-ments! This had given her the motivation she needed and Christine had religiously followed my LCD for eight weeks. To my amazement Christine's blood pressure was now completely normal at 125/75 which is phenomenal considering it had been through the roof just eight weeks ago. She was more impressed by the fact that she had lost 29 pounds and felt energetic and even tempered.

After I had examined her I said, Wow!, this is fantastic, I'm going to talk about you on my radio show this Sunday to let everyone know just how powerful the LCD is. After this radio show we had over one hundred inquiries for the diet. I have had other patients reduce their blood pressure, even with only modest weight loss in the early stages of the LCD, so that I have come to understand that healthy liver func-tion is vitally important if you are trying to reduce your blood pres-sure. I now recommend the LCD for all my patients with **high blood pressure**.

Those with **general digestive problems** such as abdominal bloat-ing, indigestion, poor appetite, alcoholic gastritis, recurrent nausea and/or vomiting of unexplained causes, and irritable bowel syn-drome, will find this diet invaluable and usually curative. In those with **irritable bowel syndrome** the LCD may need to be modified as sufferers are unable to tolerate small seeds, nuts, and grains unless they are first passed through a grinder (a small coffee grinder or high powered blender will do). Those with irritable bowel syndrome will need to grate some of their harder salad vegetables (such as carrots and beets) and they should avoid or reduce wheat products.

Anyone with persistent gastro-intestinal symptoms should see a doctor, and preferably a specialist gastroenterologist as there is always the possibility of bowel cancer and this must be excluded before natural therapies can be relied upon exclusively.

Problems that are caused by an imbalance in the immune sys-tem will always, and often dramatically, improve with a diet that cleanses and improves the function of the liver. The most common problems to manifest when the immune system is under siege are **skin rashes, allergies such as hay fever, hives and asthma, auto-immune diseases, some types of arthritis, and the modern-day epidemic of chronic fatigue syndrome**. Orthodox medicine tends to focus on suppressing the symptoms of these diseases with drugs such as cortisone creams, tablets or inhalers, anti-inflammatory drugs, and immuno-suppressant drugs. This may be necessary in acute severe cases, but in the long term such drugs may over burden the liver whose job it is to break down these drugs into harmless metabolites. These drugs can sometimes cause liver disease. This is a paradox because diseases of the immune system will be aggravated by anything that stresses or damages the liver. This is logical because a healthy liver is needed to stop toxins, viruses, and chemicals from getting past its sinusoids where the Kupffer cells chew up these nasty invaders. The liver cells (hepatocytes) are extremely busy making sure that proteins and other foods are fully broken down before they find their way into our general circulation. If the liver is not an effective barrier, toxins and incompletely digested foods find their way into our blood stream and are carried deeper into the body where they must then be dealt with by the immune system. These toxins can then damage the cells of other body organs and the immune system and inflammation in its many forms can begin. **So we can see that although the immune system protects our body from many dangers, it is the liver that protects the immune system from overload**.

All of my patients with allergies are put on the LCD and I have had

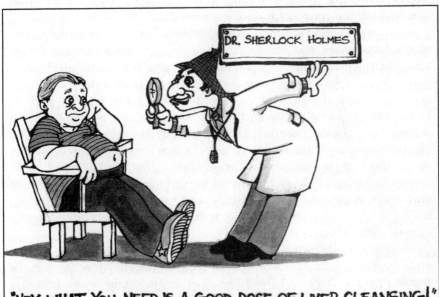

"HEY, WHAT YOU NEED IS A GOOD DOSE OF LIVER CLEANSING!"

many success stories enabling people to gradually discontinue drugs that they have previously needed to suppress allergic symptoms. Why suppress the sneeze and wheeze when one can remove the cause?

If you are taking medications for allergies such as hay fever or asthma do not discontinue them without the supervision of your local doctor because these medications can only be reduced very slowly as you gradually improve.

The vast majority of people with **chronic fatigue syndrome** (CFS) will get a big improvement after eight weeks on the LCD because if the liver is continually overworked the general energy level in the body is drained. This is wonderful news for these poor patients who have often given up hope after years of being told that there is no proven treatment for CFS, because the cause is unknown. In my experience a cause can always be found if you have a curious mind and put on your Sherlock Holmes cap—the cause is usually dietary, environmental, genetic, or stress related, and several of these factors may be acting together to make the disease worse. They all need to be addressed and in CFS patients, depression and stress will have to be treated, as well as the liver. The power of changing your diet and eating liver-friendly foods is tremendous and is the basic foundation upon which the recovery from CFS depends.

Another problem for which I am continually consulted is that of frequent **headaches and/or migraines**. Many of these patients have seen neurologists and chiropractors and have tried drug after drug; some spend nearly every day zonked out on pain killers which, of course, are toxic to the liver. Acetaminophen if taken for long periods or in high doses is particularly toxic to the liver. Not many people realize that chronic headaches can usually be greatly reduced by cleansing the liver, although Chinese doctors have long known of this association. If you suffer with headaches follow the LCD and avoid coffee and regular alcohol as these are liver toxins. Also make sure you drink 8 glasses of water daily and take magnesium 1000 mg daily. This program will gradually reduce the frequency and severity of your headaches.

Women on Hormone Replacement Therapy (HRT) often experience weight gain and/or side effects because the HRT places an extra burden on the liver. HRT induces the liver to make more proteins such as sex hormone binding globulin (SHBG) and increased clotting factors. The liver must also work harder to break down the hormones in HRT and some types of synthetic progesterone can cause increased

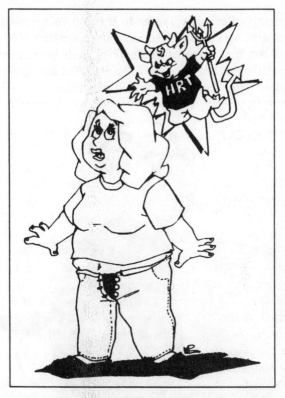

cholesterol. Oral forms of HRT are more likely to stress the liver; estrogen and progesterone patches or creams are much easier on the liver. Natural progesterone lozenges and creams are much better for the liver than synthetic progesterones. Menopausal women on HRT who are gaining weight and/or feeling tired and irritable will find that these problems will be overcome by following the LCD.

The LCD will help to repair liver damage in those who drink too much **alcohol** or those who have taken recreational drugs, especially intravenously. Those who test positive for hepatitis B and/or hepatitis C and are chronic carriers of these viruses will have less chance of developing chronic liver disease if they follow the Liver-Cleansing Diet.

Older persons will find the LCD a great tool for **increasing longevity** and vitality and staving off the degenerative diseases that unfortunately have become so common in our ageing populations. The liver definitely needs more help after the age of fifty-five, as liver weight and volume decreases with ageing. Liver blood flow decreases and the liver cells often grow larger to try and compensate. The liver becomes less able to cope with drugs, liver synthesis of proteins is reduced, and the incidence of cholesterol gallstones increases with age. To offset these changes try to follow a LCD and keep your exposure to multiple drugs and alcohol to a minimum.

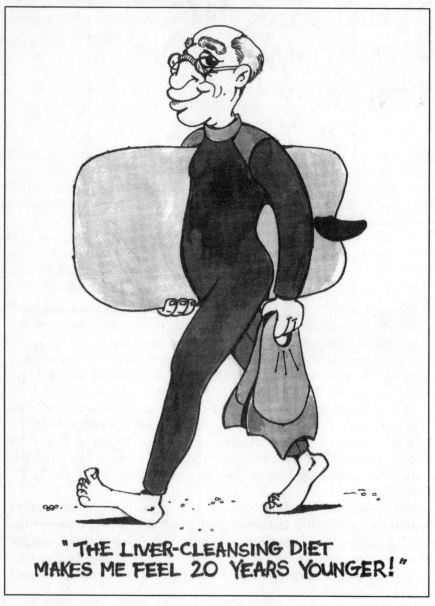

"THE LIVER-CLEANSING DIET MAKES ME FEEL 20 YEARS YOUNGER!"

Chapter 3

WHAT ARE THE SYMPTOMS OF AN UNHAPPY LIVER?

The signs of liver dysfunction vary tremendously, from very subtle symptoms to major incapacitating symptoms. In the very early stages of liver disease there are often no obvious symptoms and the problem is often discovered by accident on a routine blood test when liver enzymes are found to be elevated.

Symptoms of mild liver dysfunction may occur, even though all blood tests of liver function are "normal". The tests that doctors use routinely to check the liver are not very sensitive—they check for liver damage rather than function. Raised liver enzymes are found in blood

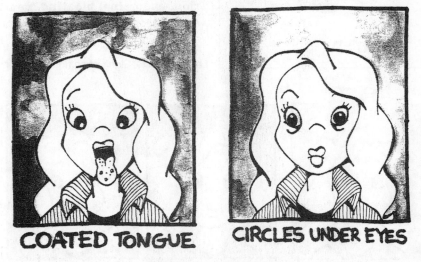

COATED TONGUE   CIRCLES UNDER EYES

Signs of an unhappy liver.

tests only after liver cells have been damaged causing them to release their intracellular enzymes. So even though the blood tests for your liver enzymes and liver proteins may be normal, this does not mean that your liver is working as well as it could or should for you to feel really well. If you have vague and non-specific symptoms for which the doctor can find no cause, I suggest that you follow my LCD as the liver is the major regulator of food energy flow in the body.

Often the first biochemical sign of liver dysfunction is raised levels of blood fats, giving readings of fasting cholesterol > 212 mg/dl and triglycerides > 177 mg/dl.

SYMPTOMS OF MILD LIVER DYSFUNCTION

Common symptoms due to poor liver function are **poor digestion**, **abdominal bloating**, **nausea** especially after fatty foods,

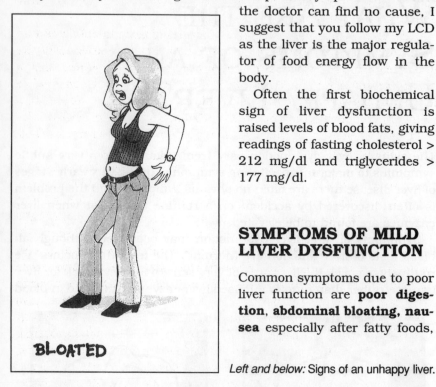

BLOATED

Left and below: Signs of an unhappy liver.

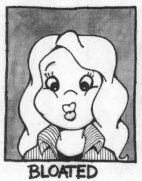
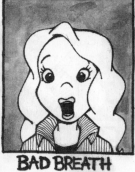

FOGGY BRAIN   BLOATED   BAD BREATH

weight gain around the abdomen, and **constipation**. So-called **"irritable bowel syndrome"** where the bowel actions are irregular and vary from diarrhea to constipation, which is associated with abdominal swelling and flatulence, is often due to a sluggish liver. If you wake up in the morning with bad breath and/or a coated tongue your liver definitely needs help. The LCD is an effective cure for these embarrassing symptoms.

If the liver is sluggish, excessive amounts of toxic metabolites find their way into the blood stream and can affect the function of the brain leading to **unpleasant mood changes, depression, and a "foggy brain"**. Your concentration and memory will not be as good as it used to be when your liver was able to maintain the correct bio-chemical composition of your blood. Patients who have followed the LCD always tell me that they feel calmer and mentally clearer as their liver function improves.

Poor liver function can trigger or exacerbate allergic conditions such as hay fever, hives, skin rashes, and asthma. This is particularly so for persons who begin to suffer with allergies for the first time in middle age and in my experience these conditions gradually improve when foods and toxins that overload the liver are eliminated. I have observed that patients with auto-immune diseases (e.g. systemic lupus erythematosus, polyarthritis, polyarteritis, and other connective tissue disorders) have often suffered with allergies prior to manifesting the symptoms of auto-immune disease. I have also noticed that in auto-immune problems the patient's diet is high in foods containing synthetic chemicals such as artificial flavorings, sweeteners, colorings and preservatives found in diet colas, candies, ice creams, packaged cookies, chips and snack foods. These chemicals build up in the liver and eventually escape the protective filtering barrier of the liver cells and flow into the blood stream. These chemicals then become incorporated into the cells of various body organs, muscles, and joints and so our own tissues gradually become "chemicalized". Our immune system can no longer recognize these chemicalized cells as a natural part of our body but instead sees them as foreign and worthy of destruction, so it produces anti-bodies to attack our own cells. This is the genesis of auto-immune disease and explains the paradox that our own immune system is fooled into attacking the very tissues it was originally designed to protect. If you suffer with an auto-immune disease you will definitely need the LCD to dechemicalize your body and reduce the irritating load upon your immune system. I have had several patients with lupus who have had a complete cure of their disease both symptomatically and by blood testing after following the LCD.

A toxic or sluggish liver can cause headaches and unfortunately the pain killers that are often required can cause a further stress on the liver, as the liver is the organ that breaks down all drugs. I have found that the LCD can be an effective preventative for a large variety of headaches including migraines, tension headaches, cluster headaches, hormonal headaches, and non-specific headaches.

Poor liver function can manifest as high blood pressure and/or fluid retention which may be difficult to control with drug therapy. This is because the liver breaks down the adrenal hormone called aldosterone. Excessive aldosterone causes retention of sodium and low potassium and these electrolyte imbalances raise the blood pressure. The liver also controls the level of blood fats and proteins and if these become excessive the blood becomes too sticky or viscous and this raises the blood pressure. I have seen the LCD bring down very high blood pressure to completely normal levels without any drugs being required. This effect is long lasting and brings a tremendous sense of relief to patients who do not want to become dependent upon anti-hypertensive drugs for the rest of their lives. High blood pressure is dangerous and increases your risk of heart attacks and strokes. The LCD can control many cases of essential hypertension and reduces the risk of cardiovascular disease which is the leading cause of death in affluent, industrialized nations. You must not stop your blood pressure medication unless your own doctor agrees to this. If you follow the eating habits espoused in my liver-cleansing program, you will eat your way to good health and longevity, in contrast to most of humanity who "dig their grave with their teeth".

The LCD is a safe and nutritious way of eating; however, if you have any medical problems such as high blood pressure or diabetes, you must not stop your medication without your own doctor's approval.

Another symptom of an unhappy liver is that of hypoglycemia or unstable blood sugar levels. This can cause wild fluctuations of blood sugar levels with very low glucose levels causing fatigue, dizziness, light headedness, and cravings for sugar. These sugar cravings are extreme and many sufferers become literally addicted to sugary things like chocolate and ice cream; they have no control over these sugar cravings, just as an alcoholic has no control once the first sip of liquor is taken. Little wonder that people with hypoglycemia

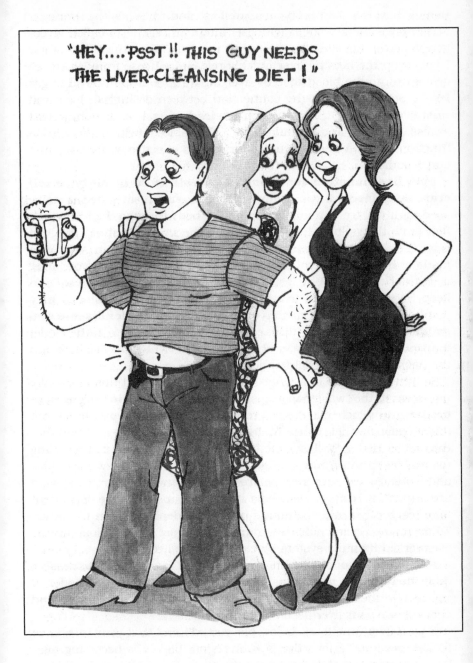

usually have a weight problem as well as candida. A healthy liver converts excess dietary sugar (glucose) into a storage form called glycogen which is kept in the liver until needed. When the blood sugar levels drop the healthy liver quickly releases glucose from its stored glycogen into the blood thereby averting a rapid drop in blood sugar levels. So one can see the connection between a sluggish liver and unstable blood sugar levels which can lead to sugar addiction, weight excess, diabetes, and candida. The LCD is able to help the liver in its function of blood glucose control and is an effective weapon against sugar addiction.

Poor liver function commonly manifests as an inability to tolerate fatty foods. If you feed your liver too much saturated or damaged fat it will try to pump it out of your body through the bile which flows into the gallbladder and then into the small intestine. This will raise the cholesterol content of your bile and can result in gallstones made of hard cholesterol and gallbladder inflammation. If your liver is not working efficiently it will not manufacture enough bile salts to keep biliary cholesterol in solution and so gallbladder stones may result. Thus poor liver function can result in **gallbladder disease and gallstones**. Gallbladder disease causes intolerance to fatty foods, nausea, vomiting, and upper abdominal pains which may radiate into the back and into the right shoulder.

Another symptom of a sluggish liver is fatigue and this is usually put down to the "wastepaper basket disease" of **chronic fatigue syndrome** into which diagnoses are thrown when tired people cannot find a cause for their ill health. In 99 per cent of such cases I find that the dietary history will give me the clue and these patients are eating too much saturated and damaged fats and not enough raw vegetables and fruits. As we have seen before, the liver and the immune system are intimately related; just like a married couple they are dependent upon each other and each one's happiness depends upon the other. To overcome chronic fatigue syndrome we must take the load off the overworked immune system by cleansing the liver.

A common symptom of an overworked or toxic liver is **excessive body heat**, which may be associated with sweating or body odor. If you feel overheated, it may not just be hot flushes or the climate, and chances are your liver needs a spring clean.

If your liver function is below par you will find that your **tolerance to alcohol** and various drugs such as antibiotics is becoming less. You may start to feel drunk after only two beers and have a bad hangover the day after only one or two drinks at the bar. You may start to become highly allergic to various prescription drugs that previously could be taken with impunity.

THE PERSPECTIVE OF CHINESE DOCTORS

In traditional Chinese medicine the liver is considered to be an extremely important organ and it is classified as one of the five main body organs, known as "zhang organs", which have a storage function. Chinese doctors teach that the smooth flow of body energy "qi" can only occur if the liver action is healthy. Many people with chronic fatigue syndrome have an underlying liver problem. The Chinese call the liver the "general of the army", in charge of body strategy and harmony. They say that although the heart stores the spirit, it is the liver that can unbalance the spirit. This can work both ways so that emotional stress can impair the functions of the liver, and disharmony in the liver can have adverse effects upon the emotional state. This can lead to irritability, anxiety, and deep depressions with suicidal tendencies. You may have heard the phrase, "He is a bit liverish today". In other words stay away as this person is in a very bad mood. The toxic liver state brought about by the abuse of alcohol or drugs will lead to not just a hangover! You will feel irritable, moody, perhaps aggressive, and definitely depressed. You may also have these symptoms if your liver is in a stagnant or sluggish state because of incorrect diet. Many cases of depression could be treated with a Liver-Cleansing Diet and liver herbs, enabling the gradual withdrawal of anti-depressant medication. The Chinese have a liver remedy with the delightful name of "the free and easy wanderer" that they use for depression and it contains the Chinese herb Xiao Yan Wan. We can all become free and easy wanderers, and slim and beautiful wanderers as well, if only we will take care of our livers; the Liver-Cleansing Diet will enable you to do this. A good liver tonic (see page 71) will also help to bring back the free and easy old you.

According to the Chinese, a stagnant liver results in "fermenting and heat" which causes "fire to rise" leading to agitation, poor sleep, dizziness, headaches and anger. The Chinese call this "gan ho". The English term "gung-ho" comes from this and describes someone who is too pushy and hyped-up. Do you feel like this sometimes? Chances are your "liver is on fire" because it is full of toxins.

The Chinese teach that the liver controls the harmonious flow of energy in the digestive tract, and if it fails to do this, too much food energy enters the stomach and spleen causing abdominal swelling and nausea. The Chinese always treat excessive weight conditions by helping liver function; however, they have had many more centuries than Western civilizations to come to this understanding.

Chinese doctors attribute poor nails and muscle and tendon stiffness to liver weakness. They also assess the state of the liver from the patient's eyes with dry, red, and itching eyes being caused from excessive heat in the liver. If your eyes are bright and clear this augurs well for your liver.

Chapter 4

LIVER PHYSIOLOGY AND FUNCTION

The liver is an extremely busy and hardworking organ as evidenced by its huge blood flow—blood passes through the liver at a rate of around 3 pints per minute.

The healthy liver is such a busy organ that its activities create a large amount of heat, increasing body temperature. That's why you will often feel hot after a large meal.

The liver is sheltered by the ribs and is tucked away in the right side of the upper abdomen. It has two anatomical parts called "lobes" and the right lobe is approximately six times larger than the left. The right and left lobes of the liver are separated by fibrous tissue known as the Falciform ligament. The large right lobe can be divided into smaller lobes called the largest right lobe proper, and the quadrate lobe and the caudate lobe, which can be seen on the underside or under surface of the liver.

As said before, the liver is the largest organ in the body so if you say to one of your friends "hey did you know that your liver is larger than your brain" you are not insulting them!

The liver is not only unique by virtue of its large size, but also by its dual blood supply. It is the only organ to have two separate sources of blood supply: the hepatic artery bringing freshly oxygenated blood from the heart and the portal vein bringing blood from the stomach and intestines which is laden with nutrients from your food.

The hepatic artery and portal vein enter the liver together through a fissure in its base called the *porta hepatis* and at this point divide into branches to supply the left and right lobes of the liver. Once

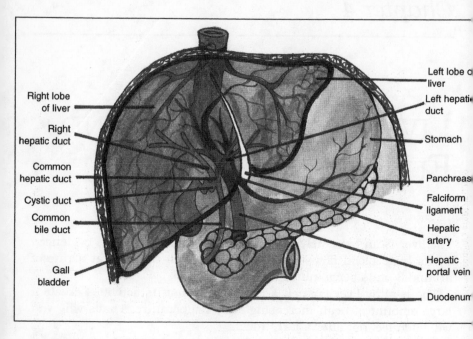

Right lobe
of liver

Right
hepatic duct

Common
hepatic duct

Cystic duct

Common
bile duct

Gall
bladder

Left lobe of
liver

Left hepatic
duct

Stomach

Panchreas

Falciform
ligament

Hepatic
artery

Hepatic
portal vein

Duodenum

Superior anterior view of the liver.

inside the liver these blood vessels keep dividing further like the
branches of a tree bringing blood to every part of the liver. These tiny
branches of blood vessels eventually empty into microscopic spaces
between the rows of liver cells. These spaces are called sinusoids and
they are vitally important for liver-cleansing and nourishment. The
sinusoidal spaces are lined by special cells such as fat storing cells,
pit cells, endothelial cells, and the most amazing cells of all—the
Kupffer cells. The Kupffer cells are highly specialized and are not easy
for your liver to replace. One could say the Kupffer cells are the trash
collection service of the liver, and we all know what happens to our
neighborhood if the local authority's trash collection service goes on
strike. Kupffer cells are mobile and look somewhat like a tiny octopus
as they travel around cleaning up the blood and lymphatic fluid
inside the sinusoid. Kupffer cells engulf and ingest dead cells, cancer
cells, yeasts, viruses, bacteria, parasites, artificial chemicals, incompletely digested or denatured proteins, and dangerous foreign particles. Once the Kupffer cell has its dangerous victim ingested, it chews

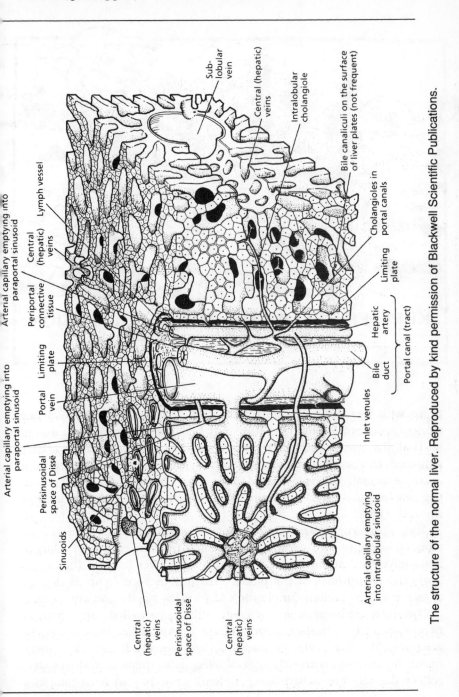

The structure of the normal liver. Reproduced by kind permission of Blackwell Scientific Publications.

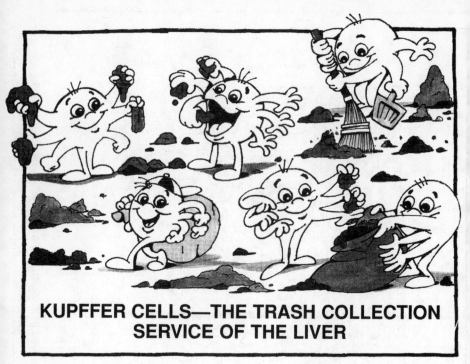

KUPFFER CELLS—THE TRASH COLLECTION SERVICE OF THE LIVER

it up with enzymes and puts it to rest. If these Kupffer cells are worked too hard for too long they may become overladen with toxins so that the liver's task of keeping your blood stream clean is not achieved. In such cases many different symptoms of poor health may occur, especially allergies, headaches, and chronic fatigue. Enter to the rescue—the Liver-Cleansing Diet which reduces the toxic load upon the liver.

After coursing in and out among the columns of liver cells, the sinusoids empty into central veins which in turn empty into larger hepatic veins that carry blood away from the liver back to the heart. Thus the cleanliness of the blood returning to your heart is dependent upon the efficient functioning of your liver cells and sinusoids.

The liver produces a yellow-green substance called bile which is necessary for the emulsification and absorption of fats from the small intestine. The liver cells produce bile and secrete it into tiny ducts which lie inbetween the clumps of liver cells; these tiny ducts that collect the bile are called bile canaliculi and they in turn join into

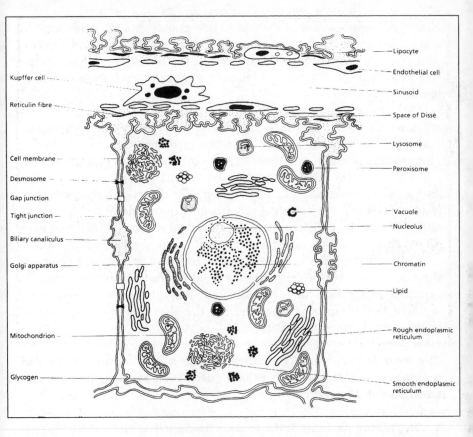

The organelles of the liver cell (hepatocyte). Reproduced by kind permission of Blackwell Scientific Publications.

larger ducts that join to form the right and left hepatic bile ducts which in turn join to form the common hepatic duct. The gallbladder is a storage sac that connects to the common hepatic duct via the cystic duct. Bile is then transported to the intestine via the common bile duct. Bile is a liquid consisting of water, bile salts, cholesterol, bile pigments, lecithin, lipids, and electrolytes. Bile salts are made by the liver cells from cholesterol which either comes from the diet or is synthesized during fat metabolism. Cholesterol itself is found in bile as a byproduct of bile-salt metabolism, but higher amounts in the bile are due to excessive saturated fats in the diet. People who eat a high-fat diet have a tendency to develop gallstones from the high amounts of cholesterol in their bile. Bile cholesterol is ideally kept in a soluble form by combining with bile salts and lecithin to form soluble particles called micelles. If there is too much cholesterol in the bile it will not be able to stay soluble and may precipitate into gallstones.

Bile salts are made from cholesterol through a sequence of chemical reactions in the liver cells so forming the primary bile acids cholic and chenodeoxycholic acids. These bile acids are combined with the amino acids taurine and glycine. This combination is called a conjugated bile acid. A bile salt is a bile acid that has lost a hydrogen ion and gained a potassium or sodium ion. Yes the production of bile in the liver is a very finely tuned process and can be deranged by a poor diet, and also by deficiencies of the amino acid taurine. All good liver tonics should contain taurine and lecithin as well as liver tonic herbs.

Bile pigments such as bilirubin give the bile a yellow-green color. If the bile ducts or liver cells are damaged so that bilirubin cannot be excreted in the bile and thus through the intestines, the bilirubin pigment builds up in the body giving the skin and eyes a yellowish color—this is called jaundice.

The liver is very versatile and performs a host of metabolic and regulatory functions. Let's take a quick look at these as they will amaze you! The liver:

1. Regulates carbohydrate metabolism—turns glucose into glycogen for storage in the liver. Liver glycogen can release glucose into the blood to maintain blood sugar levels if needed. If the body is low in carbohydrates the liver can manufacture more carbohydrates from fat or proteins.

2. Has storage functions—stores glycogen, vitamin A, vitamin D, many of the B complex vitamins, (including vitamin B_{12}) iron, and copper.

3. Regulates protein metabolism—the liver manufactures many body proteins such as albumin and blood-clotting factors such as prothrombin and fibrinogen that cause the blood to clot when needed. It makes sex hormone binding globulin which is the protein that binds the steroid sex hormones. A healthy liver is essential for a good

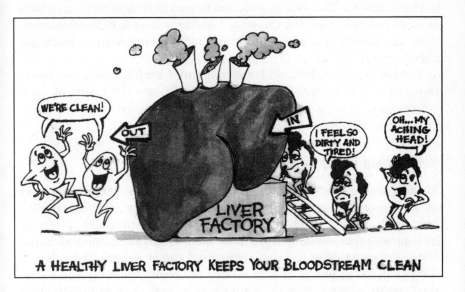

A HEALTHY LIVER FACTORY KEEPS YOUR BLOODSTREAM CLEAN

sex drive (libido) and if your liver is producing excessive amounts of the protein sex hormone binding globulin (SHBG) your libido may be poor. Many people who have followed the LCD have told me that it has improved their libido.

The liver makes many proteins for the purpose of transporting substances (such as fats, iron, hormones, and drugs) around the blood stream. One particular liver protein called high density lipoprotein (HDL) is checked frequently in blood tests as a high reading is beneficial in reducing your risk of heart disease. This is because HDL transports cholesterol out of the blood-vessel walls back to the liver for excretion. Thus a healthy liver is required for healthy blood vessels.

4. Detoxifies many toxic substances either by the Kupffer cells or by adding a chemical substance to the toxin for its elimination or deactivation. It metabolizes or biotransforms drugs, steroid hormones, and waste products of the body such as toxic ammonia. Ammonia is formed in the body from the breakdown of protein and a healthy liver is able to break it down into urea which is then excreted via the kidneys. The most important enzyme system in the liver's detoxification process is the cytochrome P-450-dependent microsmal oxidase system. Thankfully, you don't need to remember this system of liver enzymes, but it's important to know that it is highly dependent upon vitamin C and taurine and most of us don't get enough of these.

In cases of toxic overload the liver cannot keep up with detoxification requirements and thus the liver itself bears the brunt of these toxins.

SYMPTOMS OF SEVERE LIVER DISEASE

These symptoms occur only when the liver is severely damaged such as in the end stages of cirrhosis, liver cancer, or liver destruction (necrosis). This manifests as jaundice, severe depression, profound fatigue, extreme swelling of the abdomen, clumsiness, mental confusion, and coma. Bleeding can occur from the stomach or bowels and the palms of the hands may be a deep red color. There may be a flapping tremor of the hands. In such cases a liver transplant is the best solution.

The causes of severe liver disease and liver failure are alcoholism, liver cancer, analgesic abuse and overdose with the highly liver-toxic analgesic acetaminophen, severe allergic reactions to some drugs and pesticides, and infections with hepatitis B and C viruses. Thankfully, it is now possible to immunize people against hepatitis B and this should be done especially if you travel to developing countries or are a health worker. Hepatitis C virus is transmitted through blood to blood contact with someone who is already infected. This may involve drug addicts sharing needles, razor blades, unsterile skin piercing or tattooing, and needle stick injuries. It is common in persons needing repeated blood transfusions such as hemophiliacs, but the majority of hepatitis C infections occurred from transfusions given before 1990. American blood banks have screened donated blood for the hepatitis C virus since 1990. Hepatitis C contaminates blood supplies in the same way as the AIDS virus. The hepatitis C virus attacks the liver and can cause degenerative cirrhosis, liver failure, and liver cancer. The virus is proving to be a time bomb with thousands of people silently incubating the virus and it may take ten to twenty years after the initial infection before the virus causes liver disease. Only now, as those infected years ago are starting to become ill, is the true nature of hepatitis C's virulence becoming obvious.

For those who are in the early or middle stages of liver disease it is vital to follow a liver-cleansing diet and to avoid alcohol and toxic drugs. While it is important to stay under the care of a liver special-ist (hepatologist), in my opinion these specialists do not give patients enough information on diet and natural therapies for the purpose of liver regeneration. Many doctors do not believe in the power of nutri-tional medicine simply because they have never tested it or applied it to their patients. I have patients with signs and symptoms of liver disease who have been able to regenerate their liver cells and reverse liver disease with the Liver-Cleansing Diet and natural liver tonics.

THE FUTURE—ARTIFICIAL LIVERS

Artificial livers, grown from pieces of liver left over from transplant operations could save many people who currently die while waiting for a liver transplant. The revolutionary artificial liver is being devel-oped by an Anglo-German team in Birmingham UK, which has suc-cessfully cultured human liver cells outside of the body. The aim of the researchers is to use offcuts, weighing about 1–2 ounces, from human livers to grow artificial livers weighing about 16 ounces. The average adult human liver weighs around 53 ounces (3 pounds 5 ounces); however, people can survive with a much smaller liver.

The artificial liver will consist of a thick 8–inch-diameter disc of cul-tured liver cells which will receive the patient's filtered blood from a tube in the groin. A fine network of tiny permeable plastic tubes will feed the patient's blood into the cells of the artificial liver. Inside this liver the patient's blood will be detoxified, proteins will be manufac-tured, fats will be broken down, and metabolism will be restored. After this work is done, another network of tiny permeable tubes will receive the processed blood and return it to the patient's body.

Experts are watching the Birmingham project with interest. Professor Sir Roy Calne, who performed Europe's first liver transplant operation twenty-eight years ago, agrees that experiments where a healthy liver is put alongside a failing liver have proved the failing liver can regenerate. This is because the artificial liver takes the work load off the diseased liver allowing it to rest and regenerate.

Although this research is in the early stages, the ultimate aim is to make a device which could take over the entire liver function, includ-ing the manufacture of bile. In the meantime the artificial liver disc is not expected to be available until 1999.

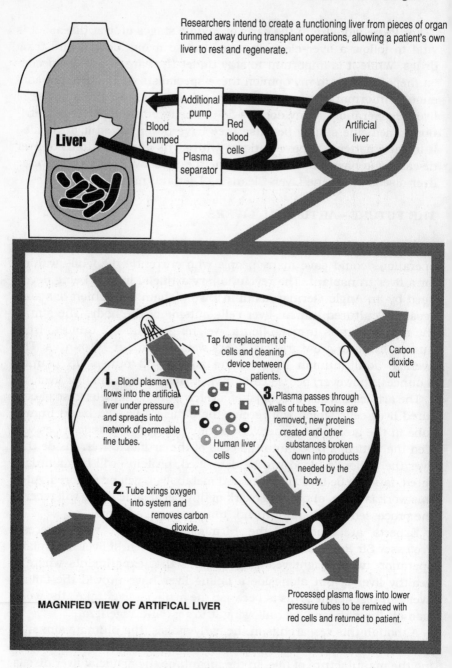

Researchers intend to create a functioning liver from pieces of organ trimmed away during transplant operations, allowing a patient's own liver to rest and regenerate.

Liver

Additional pump

Blood pumped

Red blood cells

Plasma separator

Artificial liver

Tap for replacement of cells and cleaning device between patients.

Carbon dioxide out

1. Blood plasma flows into the artificial liver under pressure and spreads into network of permeable fine tubes.

Human liver cells

3. Plasma passes through walls of tubes. Toxins are removed, new proteins created and other substances broken down into products needed by the body.

2. Tube brings oxygen into system and removes carbon dioxide.

MAGNIFIED VIEW OF ARTIFICAL LIVER

Processed plasma flows into lower pressure tubes to be remixed with red cells and returned to patient.

New liver grown from human cells.

Chapter 5

THE TWELVE **VITAL** PRINCIPLES TO IMPROVE YOUR LIVER FUNCTION

ONE

Listen to your body—don't eat if you are not hungry, have a raw juice, a piece of fruit, a small raw vegetable salad, or a glass of water instead. This applies even at meal times when you are on the LCD.

Conversely, don't put up with hunger pains—if unfulfilled they can lead to an ulcer or hypoglycemia. Far too many people place their meal times around the clock, and will eat at say 8 a.m., 1 p.m., and 7 p.m., come rain or shine, appetite or not. It's much healthier to place your meal times around your hunger in the same way that children do, and pay little heed to the clock. If you are in the habit of eating regular meals when you are not hungry, your liver will be working far too hard and will basically suffer with excessive wear and tear just like arthritic joints that are overused.

Many people, especially those who grew up during the post–Second World War depression years were made to feel guilty if they did not finish eating everything on their plate, even after their hunger was fully satisfied. For the well-being of your liver it is much better to stop eating the food on your plate once you begin to feel full and no longer have an appetite.

I suggest that you stop "thrashing your liver" into an early state of exhaustion and you will add many years to your life.

TWO

Drink at least eight to twelve glasses of filtered water daily as this helps to cleanse the liver and kidneys and aids with weight loss. Your body requires small and frequent sips of water otherwise your cells shrink with dehydration and their membranes dry out. How do your

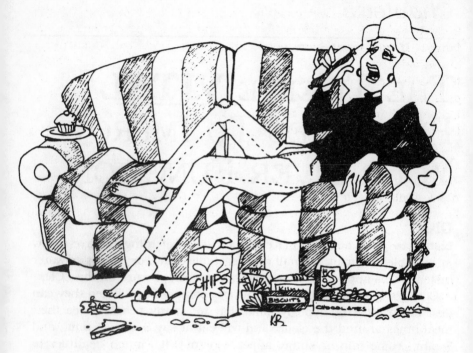

plants look if you forget to water them? Tired and wilted, and that is how your cells look under the microscope after going without sufficient water. By drinking adequate water you will reduce your chances of degenerative diseases. There is a higher incidence of Alzheimer's disease in people who do not drink water. Drink water continually throughout the day and avoid large amounts of fluid with meals.

THREE
Avoid eating large amounts of sugar, especially refined sugars, as the liver will convert this into fat.

Excessive refined sugars will be converted into fats such as cholesterol, and especially triglycerides, which can build up inside our cells causing fatty degeneration of organs (such as the liver, heart, muscles, kidneys, arteries) or will be transported to fatty areas such as the thighs, buttocks, and abdomen for storage. Eventually the blood triglycerides become too high and this is associated with an increased risk of cardiovascular disease.

Avoid all artificial sweeteners found in diet colas and some diabetic foods as these are toxic to the liver and cause hypoglycemia and fatigue. **If you must have something sweet** use fresh raw fruits, sun-dried fruits, honey, or blackstrap molasses. Refined sugar and flour cause the liver to work much harder and often result in the overgrowth of unfriendly bacteria and fungi (e.g. candida) in the body. Unrefined honey contains natural antibiotic substances that inhibit the growth of these unfriendly organisms. To observe the difference between natural unrefined honey and jams or jellies made with sugar, take a jar of each, remove their lids, and leave them on the shelf for one week. You will find that the honey remains uncontaminated while the jam is covered with a thriving culture of unhealthy fungi. A similar result occurs in your intestines. I advise you to avoid jams, jellies and sweet preserves while on the LCD.

If you are a real chocoholic try the chocolate-like alternative of carob which is found in the health food store. Carob looks, feels, and tastes like chocolate but is much healthier! It is made from the long pods of the carob tree and is particularly nice as a coating for rice cake biscuits.

Another sweet treat found at health food stores is halvah which is made from sesame seeds, honey and vanilla flavoring and may have added almonds and dried fruit. Dried fruits and raw nuts make a tasty and filling sweet treat as do natural licorice sticks from the health food store.

If you love sweet dairy ice cream then don't despair—although you cannot have dairy ice cream on the LCD, you may have a fruit sorbet which is fruit based or any other fruit ice. Put this in an ice cream cone and you will not know the difference. "Ice cream" made from soya beans may also be available and is acceptable on the liver-cleansing diet.

However, remember that although these things contain natural sugars, they are still harmful to the liver if eaten in excessive amounts or if you binge on them, in which case the liver will convert them to fat. One great advantage of the LCD is that after you have been on it for a few weeks your cravings for sugar will naturally diminish.

FOUR
Don't become obsessed with measuring calories as this is not the aim of the LCD. If you stick to the foods and meal plans in the LCD

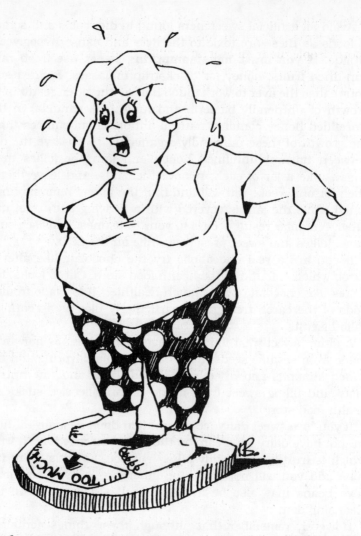

your liver function will gradually improve and weight loss will follow accordingly. Many people find that they cannot stick to a diet because the mental energy required to measure each portion of food and count the calories is too great. There is no calorie counting on the LCD as I have done all the hard work for you by ensuring that the menus are nutritionally balanced and contain sufficient calories for the average moderately active adult. If you are over sixty or you are not active, or if you feel the meals are too large for you, please feel free to reduce the size of the food portions according to your individual desires.

Simply stick to the liver-friendly foods found in the LCD and you cannot go wrong, provided you listen to your real physical hunger. Far more people die from overeating than undereating, so err on the side of eating less once your hunger is satisfied.

Ignore the bathroom scales as the aim of the LCD is to cleanse your body and rejuvenate your entire metabolism, not merely to lose weight. Weight loss will occur hand in hand with the improvement in liver function over the eight-week period of the LCD. Why stress yourself by noticing how quickly or slowly weight loss occurs? The rate of weight loss will vary considerably between different people and different age groups and if you compare yourself to a friend who may be on the diet with you, there is a good chance that you will become frustrated. During any period of dieting, weight loss may enter a temporary standstill; this phase is known as a weight loss PLATEAU and may last from two to six weeks. During the plateau phase the LCD is still working, even though weight loss is not occurring because the intracellular metabolic changes that must first occur before weight loss can recommence are taking place during the plateau phase; be patient and weight loss will resume with increased vigor. If you ignore the bathroom scales or, better still, give them to an enemy, you won't even notice this temporary plateau and will avoid frustration and give yourself a greater chance of hanging in there on the LCD for much longer.

FIVE
Avoid foods that you may be allergic to or that you know from past experience upset you. If you have a weak digestive system and feel bloated and heavy after a meal you can take digestive enzyme tablets at the *beginning* of meals. Digestive enzyme tablets or powders contain pepsin, bromelains, glutamic acid hydrochloride, papain, and pancreatic extracts and some people find them very helpful. Another tip for those with weak digestion is to always begin each meal with something raw; for example, begin breakfast with one or two pieces of raw fruit and lunch and dinner with a raw vegetable salad. These raw foods contain living enzymes which will supplement your own enzymes to enhance digestion. Always chew your food slowly and thoroughly as digestion begins with saliva mixed with food in the mouth. As people age, the production of hydrochloric acid from the stomach often becomes inadequate for efficient digestion of proteins and this can be overcome by sipping a small glass of water containing one teaspoon of

apple cider vinegar during every meal. The most common foods to cause intestinal irritation and irritable bowel syndrome are wheat and dairy products (milk, butter, cheese, cream, ice cream, chocolate). This is because wheat and dairy products contain reactive proteins as well as gluten and lactose and many people feel much less bloated when they avoid these foods completely. Don't overdose on coffee as excessive amounts are toxic for the liver. While on the LCD restrict coffee to no more than one to two cups a day or better still avoid it completely. Real natural coffee from freshly ground coffee beans is healthier than instant coffee. If you use decaffeinated coffee make sure that you avoid brands in which chemicals are used to remove the caffeine.

SIX

Be aware of good intestinal hygiene as the liver must filter out and destroy any bacteria and viruses present in our food. If we present the liver with too many unfriendly organisms or dangerous bacteria, such as salmonella or shigella, these infectious agents may invade our blood stream making us seriously ill. They may also permanently damage the liver. To reduce this risk only eat foods that are fresh and avoid the regular reheating of food as bacteria breed in stored cooked foods, especially meats. Never reheat food more than once. Avoid fast food and takeout food, especially meat, as it may not be fresh. Always wash your hands before eating. Avoid foods containing uncooked eggs, unless you are certain the eggs have been stored under refrigeration. When travelling in under-developed countries avoid unpeeled fruits and vegetables, raw foods and shell fish, such as oysters, as these may be contaminated with many different organisms capable of causing gastroenteritis. It is wise to avoid salads while overseas unless you can make them yourself, as in under-developed countries they may be washed in the local water supply which can cause gastroenteritis. Also, drinking water should be boiled or come in sealed bottles (carbonated is safest).

Many packaged and processed foods found on supermarket shelves are kept "consumable" only because they are laden with preservatives and yet they are still full of unfriendly organisms in a dormant state. As soon as this type of processed and preserved food hits your intestines, the preservatives wear off and the bugs begin to grow inside you. We have seen cases of severe food poisoning from the consumption of preserved delicatessen meats such as, Italian sausage, ham, smoked meats, sausages, frankfurters, corned beef, bacon, and pizza meats and in some instances these infections can be fatal. All those on a liver-cleansing program are better to avoid these types of preserved meats which place high digestive and bacterial loads upon the liver.

SEVEN
Do not eat if you feel stressed or anxious as during these states your blood flow is diverted away from the intestines and liver to other areas of the body. Eating at these times will lead to abdominal bloating and poor digestion.

EIGHT
Check if organically grown fresh produce free of pesticides is available in your area. Your local health food store will know and you can often have these things home delivered from a food co-operative. Ask your butcher if organically reared products are available and always buy free-range eggs and chickens. These type of products contain less pesticides, hormones, antibiotics, and saturated fat. Buy products containing natural ingredients and avoid processed foods containing artificial chemicals such as preservatives, colorings, flavorings and artificial sweeteners. To do this you will need to shop more at the fruit market, fish market, butcher, and health food store and less at the supermarket, although many large food chains are beginning to include health sections containing natural products free of artificial chemicals.

NINE
Obtain your protein from diverse sources (including legumes), not just from animal products such as meat, eggs, and fish. The LCD does contain some chicken (preferably free range), fish, and eggs; however, there are also many meals in which protein is obtained from legumes, grains, cereals, nuts, and seeds. You can obtain first-class protein by combining any three of the four following foods—grains, nuts, seeds, and legumes, at one meal. First-class protein from these sources is just as complete as protein from animal products and contains all of the eight essential amino acids. Grains are wheat, buckwheat, rice, barley, rye, oats, millet, spelt, kamut, quinoa, amaranth, and there are others that your health food store may stock. If you have irritable bowel syndrome or intestinal allergies you may find that wheat produces a bad reaction and in such cases rice is a well-tolerated alternative. Legumes, also known as pulses are

beans (such as soya beans, adzuki beans, butter beans, lima beans, kidney beans, etc.), peas, chickpeas, and lentils and they provide valuable protein, essential fatty acids, fiber, plant hormones, calcium, iron, magnesium, zinc, and B vitamins. In general people do not eat enough legumes, perhaps because they find them too difficult to prepare, so here are some tips to make them simple and easy to digest. Use only good quality beans and discard any that are shrunken or discolored. Rinse them in a sieve and soak them overnight for 12 to 24 hours—you will need four measures of water to one measure of beans. Some beans, such as soya beans, are best cooked in a pressure cooker. Place the beans in a large pan with a water level 2 inches above the beans and bring them quickly to the boil, removing any discolored scum which floats to the top. Keep the beans simmering, not boiling, and well covered with water. Continue cooking until the beans can easily be broken with a sharp knife. If you are too busy it is acceptable to use canned legumes and there are many to choose from such as baked beans, chickpeas, soya beans, chili beans, red kidney beans, three and four bean mix, butter beans, and lentils. If the canned beans have sauces containing lots of salt and sugar, rinse this off with water before using them in the LCD recipes. Legumes can also be sprouted for use in salads. This is easy to do at home on a windowsill or in an airy cupboard, in a sprouting tray found at supermarkets and health food stores. Sprouting legumes and seeds greatly increases their nutritional and liver-cleansing properties because the sprouting process increases their content of vitamin C, amino acids, and fatty acids. Alternatively, you can easily purchase sprouted legumes and seeds at supermarkets and health food stores, but make sure they are fresh and not moldy.

Seeds are an excellent source of essential fatty acids, protein, plant hormones, and fiber and are part of the LCD. I recommend linseeds, sunflower, sesame, and pumpkin seeds. For most people they are best put through a coffee grinder or high powered blender to produce a fine powder, otherwise they can be indigestible. An excellent way to boost your essential fatty acids and protein is to make a mixture of linseeds (flaxseeds), sunflower seeds, and almonds (called LSA) by passing them through a grinder to make a fine, delicious, sweet, and nutty tasting powder to sprinkle on your fruit, vegetables, cereal or to add to one of the health shakes in the LCD. You should use three measures of linseeds, two measures of sunflower seeds, and one measure of almonds. If you use this regularly you will never suffer from constipation. In really stubborn cases of constipation add two to three tablespoons of psyllium husks to the LSA mixture everyday. LSA is also a great "brain food" and will help those with a poor memory!

Nuts are very rich in unsaturated oils and should only be eaten fresh and raw. If they have been shelled for a long time and exposed to the air this will have caused their oils to become rancid and no longer beneficial. Buy nuts that are in sealed bags with a use-by date or nuts still in their shells. If you are using combinations of legumes, seeds, nuts, and cereals as a protein source it is best not to eat them with meat or eggs if you have a weak digestive system.

TEN

Choose your breads and spreads wisely. It is important to eat only good quality breads on the LCD. These breads provide fiber, minerals, and B vitamins. In the good old days bread was made by the local baker using simple ingredients of flour, water, yeast, and salt. Today, most supermarket breads are made with mass production methods using ingredients like hydrogenated vegetable oils, potassium bromate, disodium dihydrogen diphosphate, monoacetyltartaric acid, azodicarbonamide, and other artificial chemicals that must be dealt with by your overworked liver. Larger amounts of yeast, rapid fermentation processes, and "improvers" found in these mass-produced breads can cause bloating and irritable bowel syndrome. Supermarket "brown" breads may be just white breads colored with artificial caramel. So when on the LCD I suggest you go to the health food store to buy breads free of artificial chemicals. If you have irritable bowel syndrome use stone ground breads which have a fine texture and are free of little grainy bits. Vary the types of breads you eat to reduce allergies—try rye, wheat, corn, oats, rice, barley, and others available in health food stores. For something lighter try rice crackers, rye crackers or yeast-free pita bread. If you are allergic to yeast try yeast-free breads or a sourdough loaf.

While on the LCD it is essential that you avoid margarine and/or butter as a spread on your breads. If you are trying to lose weight it will be an uphill and frustrating battle if you continue to use these as spreads. After a few weeks, you won't even miss them! If you are one of those bread lovers who must have a spread there are three spread alternatives that you may use on the LCD. These are fresh avocado, hummus, or tahini which contain natural essential fatty acids friendly to the liver. Tahini paste is made from sesame seeds and is high in minerals, especially calcium. Hummus is a paste made from chick-peas, sesame seeds and garlic and gives your bread a nice savory taste for sandwiches. Experiment with these three spreads and you will have plenty of variety. When you use hummus or tahini as a spread on your bread you also have a good source of protein. You can make your own hummus (see recipe page 147) or buy hummus and tahini from the health food store or supermarket.

ELEVEN

Avoid constipation by eating plenty of **raw** fruits and vegetables and drinking water throughout the day. You can make your own nutritious high-fiber breakfast muesli from linseeds, pepitas, sunflower seeds, sesame seeds, psyllium husks, oat bran, rice bran, and lecithin granules. Use one cup of each and this will last you four weeks. Pass all the seeds through a grinder first or ask your health food store to make it up for you. By avoiding constipation you will avoid the growth of unfriendly organisms in your large bowel. To increase the amount of the friendly acidophilus and lactobacilli bacteria in your bowel you may take powdered forms of these bacteria or eat soya-bean yogurts. If you are really keen you can buy a yogurt-making machine and make your own yogurt from soya milk. One of my patients does this and told me that yogurt-making machines are readily available at very reasonable prices. Use 1 quart of warm soya milk and add three tablespoons of any unflavored acidophilus and bifidus yogurt for the culture. On the LCD we want you to avoid all dairy products including cows' milk yogurt.

I have found that many patients with constipation also have dyspepsia, heartburn, reflux and indigestion. I have included all these terms because they are often used interchangeably. If you have these complaints avoid regular consumption of antacid medications containing the toxic metal aluminium. Instead use safer antacids containing calcium carbonate, magnesium carbonate, aloe vera juice and the herbs chamomile, meadowsweet, golden seal, peppermint and slippery elm.

TWELVE

Avoid excessive saturated or damaged fats as these will harm your liver if you eat them regularly. These unhealthy fats can cause liver damage with chances of a "fatty liver", similar to that seen in heavy alcohol consumption.

Many weight watchers try to follow a completely fat-free diet, believing that this will speed up weight loss; however, if this is done for more than four weeks, symptoms of essential fatty acid deficiency will start to occur. Furthermore, if you completely exclude healthy fats, namely essential fatty acids, from your diet your liver function and metabolism will slow down leading to easy weight gain! Symptoms of essential fatty acid deficiency are: dry and itchy skin, eczema, hair loss, joint pains, reduced fertility, increased rate of miscarriage, depression and poor memory, slow metabolic rate with weight gain, reduced immune function, hormonal imbalances, liver degeneration, fatigue, circulatory problems, degenerative diseases, increased rate of ageing, and high triglycerides. Obviously, these healthy essential fatty acids are vital for normal human metabolism and you definitely don't want to be deficient in them.

I see thousands of overweight people and I always take a detailed dietary history of exactly what the patient eats on an average day. I always find that the balance of fats in their diets is unfavorable for healthy liver function and I try to eliminate the unhealthy fats from their diets. Many of these overweight patients do not eat excessive amounts of food or calories; their problems are due solely to the consumption of the wrong type of fats that place heavy burdens upon the liver. The liver is the supreme fat-burning organ of the body, if you choke it with damaged fats it will be unable to perform its metabolic functions and your entire metabolism will slow down. As a result you will gain weight easily particularly around the abdominal area. The liver takes excessive dietary fat and turns it into cholesterol which it then turns into bile which is pumped out of your body through the intestines. Provided your diet is high in fiber this excess fat will pass through you via your bowel actions. Thus, in a simplistic way we could say that a healthy liver pumps fat out of your body and thus keeps you slim. The LCD stimulates this fat eliminating process and makes it much easier to lose those stubborn fat deposits, even in people who have been overweight for years.

A healthy liver also manufactures a specialized coating for fat called lipoprotein which enables fat to travel around in the blood stream. If your liver cannot do this efficiently fat builds up in the liver causing a "fatty liver" and once this occurs it becomes increasingly difficult to lose weight. Eating the wrong foods for your liver will cause an imbalance in the liver's production of lipoproteins so that you will have too much low-density lipoprotein (LDL) and not enough high-density lipoprotein (HDL). This situation will increase your risk of atherosclerosis, heart disease, stroke, and high blood pressure. So now you can see that a healthy liver is needed to reduce your risk of cardiovascular disease which is by far the leading cause of death in affluent, industrialized populations.

The type of fats you eat on a daily basis is so important to your health and longevity and will have the greatest influence of all upon your liver function and weight. Therefore, we should take a look at the good and the bad fats in more detail.

UNDERSTANDING DIETARY FATS

HEALTHY FATS
These are called essential fatty acids (EFAs) for two reasons:

1. They are essential in the diet as the body cannot manufacture them
2. They are essential for health

Essential fatty acids are the major constituents of the membranes around the outside of our cells and also the tiny metabolic organs inside every cell (see diagram page 39). Without sufficient EFAs our cell walls and the cell's internal organs develop holes and become prone to leakage and poor energy transfer. Little wonder that our metabolism slows down and weight gain occurs. EFAs also enable the cell membrane to eliminate toxins from the inside to the outside of the cell and are vital for your liver cells (hepatocytes and Kupffer cells) to cleanse the blood of toxic material. EFAs keep your cell barriers strong and thus improve the efficiency of the immune system.

Lets take a look at the names and sources of these desirable EFAs.

OMEGA 6 EFAs

Linoleic Acid (LA) and Gamma-Linolenic Acid (GLA)
These unsaturated EFAs are most beneficial and are found in saf-flower seeds, sunflower seeds, hemp seeds, flaxseed (linseed), sesame seeds, pumpkin seeds, walnuts, soya beans, evening primrose oil,

Table of Sources and Functions of Fatty Acids

This table provides an overview of selected fatty acids, together with the types of prostaglandins they are used to produce, the effects of these prostaglandins on the body, and food sources of the fatty acids. The correct balance of fatty acids—specifically, more omega-3 and omega-6 essential fatty acids and less arachidonic acid—is needed to create the optimal balance of prostaglandins in the body.

Prostaglandin Family Produced From These Fatty Acids	Actions of These Prostaglandins in the Body	Food Sources of These Fatty Acids
OMEGA-6 ESSENTIAL FATTY ACIDS **LINOLEIC ACID AND GAMMA-LINOLENIC ACID**		
PG_1 (desirable)	Reduce pain and inflammation; improve skin; increase energy and vitality.	Breast milk; sesame, safflower, cotton, and sunflower seeds and oil (cold-pressed); corn and corn oil; soybeans; raw nuts; legumes; leafy greens; black currant seeds; and their oil; evening primrose oil; borage oil; gooseberry oil; spirulina; soybeans; lecithin.
OMEGA-3 ESSENTIAL FATTY ACIDS **ALPHA-LINOLENIC ACID AND EICOSAPENTAENOIC ACID(EPA)**		
PG_3 (desirable)	Reduce pain and inflammation; help circulation.	Fresh fish from cold, deep oceans (such as mackerel, tuna, herring, sablefish, flounder, sardines, salmon); rainbow trout; bass. Fish must not be fried. Also, linseed oil; black currant and pumpkin seeds and their oil; cod liver oil; shrimp; oysters; leafy greens; canola oil; soybeans; walnuts; wheat germ; wheat sprouts; fresh sea vegetables; fish oil capsules.
OMEGA-6 *NON*ESSENTIAL FATTY ACID **ARACHIDONIC ACID (AA)**		
PG_2 (undesirable)	Excess amounts may increase pain and inflammation and can result in excessively sticky blood platelets	Animal meats; whole-milk dairy products; preserved meats; fried foods; processed and takeout foods; coconut and palm oils.

borage oil (star flower oil), black currant seed oil, spirulina, and lecithin. Another Omega 6 EFA called Dihomogamma-Linolenic Acid (DGLA) is found in human breast milk. Many people, especially those with poor liver function, do not get enough of these Omega 6 EFAs in their diets and there can be a significant variation in requirements for optimal health between individuals, especially in those with chronic diseases. The daily requirement for Omega 6 EFAs can vary from 3 to 18 grams daily. The LCD will give you sufficient Omega 6 EFAs and you will obviously need a good grinder. An inexpensive coffee grinder will do the job very well, and you may snack on these seeds if you get peckish.

OMEGA 3 EFAS

Alpha Linolenic Acid (LNA) and Eicosapentaenoic Acid (EPA) and Docosahexaenoic Acid (DHA)

These unsaturated EFAs are just as beneficial as those of the Omega 6 group and many people do not obtain enough of these from their diet for optimal health. LNA is found in flaxseeds (linseeds), hemp seeds, canola, soya beans, walnuts, pumpkin seeds, chia and kukui (candle nut oils), and dark green leafy vegetables. EPA and DHA are found in cold water fish and marine animals such as sardines, tuna, trout, mackerel, and salmon. Chinese snake oil also gets its healing properties from its Omega 3 EFA content.

Certain organs of land animals such as adrenal glands and brains are also high in DHA and EPA but we do not recommend these delicacies on the LCD.

Other beneficial fatty acids that are monounsaturated can be obtained from avocados, fresh unshelled peanuts, almonds, macadamia nuts, cashew nuts, pecan nuts, and olive oil. All these nuts must be eaten fresh if their oils are to be beneficial.

OILS AIN'T OILS

You now understand which foods and oils can provide your body with EFAs that are vital for healthy metabolism and the prevention of degenerative diseases. However, it is vitally important for you to understand that these oils are only beneficial if they are eaten in their natural states and not damaged by the elements or processing. This is because **EFAs are very vulnerable** to deterioration from exposure to **light, air or heat.**

Sunlight or artificial light will cause free radical production in the oils whereas the air's oxygen will cause oxidation of the EFAs breaking them down so that the oil becomes rancid. When oils become rancid their EFAs are oxidized to dangerous polymers, hydroperoxyaldehydes, and peroxides which can place increased burdens upon the liver and immune system and damage cell membranes.

The application of heat destroys EFAs by twisting their molecules into an abnormal straighter new shape called a "trans-shape". This occurs during the hydrogenation process and also when we fry oils at high temperatures (especially deep frying with reheated oils as can occur in some takeouts). Deep-fried and/or repeatedly reheated oils contain many toxic fats such as toxic cyclic monomers which can lead to fatty livers in experimental animals and diseases in humans such as atherosclerosis, reduced immune function, poor cellular oxygenation, and an increased risk of cancer. Try not to eat deep-fried foods on a regular basis, and if you have a sluggish liver or gall-bladder disease NEVER eat deep-fried foods.

Hydrogenation is used to turn natural oils into unhealthy trans-fatty acids for processed oils, margarines and shortenings used in convenience foods, and baked goods such as cookies and cakes. The trans-fatty acids in margarines and other hydrogenated vegetable oils are straight in shape which enables these products to stay solid at room temperature. They may be spreadable and easier to use than liquid oils but as far as your body is concerned they are not easy to use at all because they are not easily biodegradable. I call them "plastic fats" because they are not really natural or organic as far as our metabolism is concerned.

In natural oils the EFAs are called cis-fatty acids and they are curly and bent in shape which keeps the oil liquid. During heating or hydrogenation these cis-fatty acids are twisted into a straighter trans-fatty acid with its head on backwards. Once these distorted trans-fatty acids get into our bodies they cause some confusion for our cells because with their strange shape they do not quite fit into the biological systems of our cells—call them social misfits in cellular society. Trans-fatty acids cause big problems for our cell membranes because they do not fit correctly into the membrane which results in holes and electrical short circuits in the membrane. This reduces the protective quality of the membrane and impairs its energy transfer and elimination functions. Trans-fatty acids not only cause problems for the membranes around the outside of our cells, they also cause the same problems for the membranes inside the cell such as the mitochondria and other tiny organelles (see diagram page 39). This impairs the enzyme systems and energy production inside the cell.

Trans-fatty acids are bad news for your liver because they impair the function of the liver's most important detoxification enzyme system called the Cytochrome P 450 enzymes. The Cytochrome P 450 liver enzymes break down toxins and carcinogens.

Trans-fatty acids are "stickier" than natural cis-fatty acids which makes your blood platelets more sticky and can result in increased blood clots and poor blood flow in tiny blood vessels.

It is easy to understand how sluggish metabolism and poor health can result when our cells attempt to use the distorted molecules of trans-fatty acids for their vital functions and structures. If we eat large amounts of these damaged fats for a long time the consequences can be serious. Adverse effects upon the liver and heart (such as fatty degeneration of these organs) may occur and the immune system may function abnormally.

Many people believe that margarines and other processed vegetable oils are healthy and have been designed to be superior to animal fats. I believe this is misleading—they are not. Indeed, excess trans-fatty acids will be converted by the body into cholesterol and triglycerides which can increase cardiovascular disease. In 1990 the *New England Journal of Medicine* published the results of a large study which showed that trans-fatty acid consumption increased total cholesterol and undesirable low-density lipoprotein fats and these are known risk factors for cardiovascular disease.

So by now you probably view margarines, French fries and chips, and packaged cookies with sheer terror. If so, my mission has worked, as I don't want you to eat these things on a regular basis. Trans-fatty acids have adverse effects upon the immune system, cardiovascular system, fat metabolism, liver function, cell membranes, and the production of body energy.

Consider margarines, hydrogenated and partially hydrogenated vegetable oils, shortenings, and shortening oils as veritable liver foes. They are definitely out during the eight-week Liver-Cleansing Diet.

When you are not on the LCD I suggest that you keep your consumption of these damaged fats to a minimum, although I too am human and realize that you cannot be perfect all the time. One of the ladies who works with me in the Women's Health Advisory Service has a penchant for French fries and disappears every Wednesday lunch time with a sneaky grin on her face. Ten minutes later, in she comes with her white grease-stained packet of French fries and everyone (except me, of course!) sneaks a few from her. She is a little android-shaped woman with a cuddly pot belly and really loves her food which was obvious when I first met her ten years ago. At this time she was very overweight and suffered with high blood pressure and arthritis. Today she is in much better form because she has increased the amounts of raw vegetables, fish, and grains in her diet and the healthy fats found in these foods have enabled her to have her occasional special treats without the return of obesity and high blood pressure.

TAKE CARE OF YOUR OILS

Dietary oils will only take care of us if we take care of them by reducing their exposure to air, heat, and light. Natural food oils such as those contained in fish, seeds, nuts, avocados, olives, and legumes are protected from light, air, and heat by virtue of the skins, coverings, and shells around them and as such are fresher and healthier than the bottled versions of their contained oils. However, for salad dressings, home-made cakes, and light stir frying you will need some good quality oil that tastes pleasant. Ideally you should buy unrefined oils that have been mechanically pressed (genuinely cold-pressed) and kept in dark-colored glass bottles to block out the light. Keep your bottle of oil in the fridge. Sometimes these high quality oils can be harder to find, but your health food store should be able to help. **Virgin olive oil** is generally available and is a good choice because it is made commercially with mechanical pressing and has not been heated, refined or bleached—please pay that little bit extra to get **virgin** olive oil.

Oily fish should be eaten freshly cooked or canned and not deep fried or smoked. During deep frying or the smoking process the EFAs in the fish will be damaged and oxidized. Canned or tinned fish such as salmon, tuna, sardines, and mackerel are a healthy source of oils, provided they are not smoked.

STIR-FRYING

Ideally one should never fry food in oils, especially at high temperatures. However there is a method of "stir-frying" which is acceptable but it takes more time and care. We can take a leaf out of the recipe books of traditional Chinese cooks who first put water in the wok, not oil, and then add the vegetables and after slow heating add a small amount of oil. This method keeps the cooking temperatures down to 212°F which is a nondestructive temperature and avoids overheating and oxidation. Do not put the oil in the wok first as it becomes overheated and burnt, causing destruction of its EFAs. Use only a low heat or small flame and stay by the wok to continually monitor its temperature. It is beneficial to add garlic and onions to the wok as they are rich in sulfur which minimizes free radical damage. Some oils are less damaged by heating than others and the best oils for stir frying are canola oil, sesame oil, peanut oil, high oleic sunflower and safflower oils, and olive oil.

When using this slow heating method of stir-frying don't cook the food for too long—ten minutes will usually do, and you will find that the food is crisper and has more flavor.

CHOLESTEROL

Cholesterol is a hard waxy fatty substance that is only found in foods from animal sources such as eggs, meat, dairy products, fish, and shellfish. Plant foods do not contain cholesterol. In the minds of most people cholesterol is a bad thing synonymous with blocked arteries and heart attacks. However, it is only excess cholesterol in the body that causes problems and reasonable amounts of cholesterol are vital for human metabolism. Cholesterol is needed to give cell membranes a certain amount of stiffness. The glands of the endocrine system use cholesterol as the raw material for making hormones, such as the sex hormones (estrogen, progesterone, androgens) and cortisone. Vitamin D is made from cholesterol and the liver makes bile from cholesterol. The body can make all the cholesterol it needs from dietary proteins, fats, and sugars and does not depend upon food sources of cholesterol. In other words you can be perfectly healthy even if you don't eat any foods containing cholesterol, as your body will manufacture all the cholesterol it needs if your levels get too low. The more calories you consume from protein, sugar, saturated fats, and other non-essential fatty acids the more cholesterol your body will make, so you can end up with high cholesterol levels just by eating too much, even though you may not be eating any cholesterol-containing foods.

Although your body can make cholesterol, once made, it cannot break it down, so you can see that it is easy for an excess to occur. **Cholesterol can only be removed from the body by the liver in the form of bile**. A healthy liver will pump cholesterol via the bile, out into the intestines; however, if dietary fiber is absent over 90 percent of the cholesterol and bile acids are reabsorbed from the bowel and recycled back to the liver. This form of recycling is not good for your internal environment and may cause high cholesterol levels in those on a low-fiber diet.

Doctors advise patients to keep their total cholesterol levels below 200 mg/dl and to do this you need to follow a balanced diet such as the LCD and you also need a healthy liver. Once again we tend to forget the master fat burner and regulator—the liver! As you know, if your liver is healthy it will discard excess cholesterol via the bile and pump it out into the intestines where it can be carried away in high-fiber foods through the bowel actions. **This is what all overweight people dream of—an organ to pump fat out of their body as fast as possible—just keep your liver healthy and clean and you have the key!**

You also need a healthy liver to prevent excess cholesterol in the bloodstream from being dumped into plaques on the inner lining of your blood vessels. To keep blood cholesterol in a safe form you need plenty of high density lipoproteins (HDLs) as these act as scavengers and pick up free cholesterol in the blood and carry it back to the liver to be reused or turned into bile. Lipoproteins must be manufactured by the liver as they are not found in foods and many people with a sluggish liver do not produce sufficient high-density lipoproteins (HDLs). Ask your own doctor to check your levels of HDL and hopefully they will be towards the high end of the normal range which for HDL is 35 – 65 mg/dcl. The **ratio** of total cholesterol to HDL = (total cholesterol ÷ by HDL) can be a predictor of cardiovascular disease and a ratio of 3.5, or better still even lower, is desirable; your local doctor can easily measure this for you. If your HDL is too low (say less than 35), or your CHOL/HDL ratio is too high (greater than 5.5), this is a very good reason to follow the LCD. After eight weeks on this diet ask your doctor to recheck these blood tests and you will be very pleased.

Here is an interesting story. Tony, aged fifty-five, came to see me with his wife Maria as both of them were distressed by the results of a recent blood test done on Tony by his local doctor. This had shown high cholesterol and low levels of HDL, as well as raised liver enzymes signifying liver damage. Tony had seen a gastroenterologist who specialized in liver diseases (a hepatologist) and after various tests was told that there was no cause evident for his liver malfunction. Tony was not reassured as his mother had died from some mysterious liver inflammation in her early sixties. Maria did most of the talking and chastized her husband because his diet was not as healthy as her own and she told me that Tony ate too much cheese, drank too much red wine, and did not drink water. Tony was by no stretch of the imagination an alcoholic and drank alcohol in an amount that is typical of many "healthy" men; he drank around two glasses of wine and two or three cans of beer a day. Very importantly, he did not eat many raw fruits and vegetables, but preferred hard yellow mature cheeses and Italian sausages such as cabanossi, salami, and pepperoni. Poor Tony's liver was working overtime seven days a week and was not coping. Maria and I worked out a plan of attack—Tony could have one glass of red wine daily if he would follow the LCD for eight weeks. Thanks to Maria and the fear of following in his mother's footsteps, Tony did very well in sticking to the LCD and his liver specialist was amazed to find that his liver enzymes were normal and that his cholesterol levels had reduced by several points after only eight weeks.

Many men today are similar to Tony in that they drink a little too much alcohol, eat too much saturated fat in the form of cheese and meat, don't drink enough water, and don't eat sufficient raw fruits and vegetables. By the time they get to middle age their liver is feeling tired and overburdened and their cholesterol is on the way up. The eight-week LCD is most beneficial for men in this situation who feel like their liver needs a good spring cleaning.

For those with high total cholesterol the following is recommended:
A high-fiber diet (such as the LCD) to carry cholesterol out of the body via the bowel actions. The fibers in psyllium husks and oat bran are able to lower cholesterol.

Lecithin in a daily dose of 3–4 tablespoons of the fresh lecithin granules or 4000 mg of lecithin capsules.

Lecithin keeps fats in solution by breaking them up into small droplets. It acts like a dishwashing detergent does, when you wash your greasy pots and pans. Lecithin is needed to keep cholesterol soluble and prevents it from being deposited in plaques on the inner lining of your blood vessels.

Take **anti-oxidants, especially vitamin C**, as this prevents oxidation of the fats in your bloodstream and your arterial linings. Take 1000 to 4000 mg of vitamin C daily and drink at least ten glasses of water daily. This will really help to lower cholesterol levels as well as improve liver function.

Take **garlic** capsules in a dose of 2000 to 4000 mg daily and/or eat fresh garlic and onions regularly. Odorless garlic capsules are not as good as the real thing, but they will still be able to produce a significant improvement in your cholesterol levels. Take garlic with food and include it in your cooking.

Talk to your doctor about using **vitamin B$_3$** in the form of niacin or nicotinic acid if you have elevated cholesterol levels. Vitamin B$_3$ can reduce the risk of death for those who have suffered heart attacks. Vitamin B$_3$ not only lowers cholesterol, it also detoxifies pollutants, alcohol, and some pain killer drugs. Back in the 1950s researchers described the cholesterol-lowering effects of vitamin B$_3$ and although in those days huge doses were used, nowadays good results are achieved with smaller doses ranging from 500 mg to 2000 mg daily. Always take vitamin B$_3$ at the beginning of meals and never on an empty stomach. Vitamin B$_3$ should only be prescribed under medical supervision as high doses can cause flushing and gastro-intestinal problems.

Nutritional medicine is very powerful, as well as being risk free, and I have found that 99 percent of people can control their cholesterol levels by diet alone.

Chapter 6

NATURAL THERAPIES FOR YOUR LIVER

Psyllium

Psyllium seeds come from the Indian plant, *Plantago ovata*. Psyllium is derived from the husks of psyllium seeds and is a soluble mucilloid fiber. By taking 1 level teaspoon of psyllium three times daily you can lower cholesterol levels by 14–20 per cent after eight weeks. Psyllium can reduce an excessive appetite and by mixing 1 level teaspoon of psyllium powder in a glass of juice and drinking it before meals you can feel partially full before beginning your meal.

Those with sluggish liver function often have difficulty metabolizing fats and may have high cholesterol levels. Psyllium can help in such cases.

The largest trial ever conducted into the effects of psyllium fiber carried out at the Universities of Newcastle and Sydney in Australia has proven that it is probably the best cholesterol-lowering fiber available. Psyllium is proving a more consistent cholesterol-lowering agent than oat fiber. Psyllium is a plentiful source of soluble fiber, and it is well accepted that soluble fiber has a significant role in the prevention and treatment of elevated cholesterol levels. Psyllium is best taken at the beginning of meals.

Taurine

Taurine, one of the lesser-known amino acids, plays several important roles in the body and is an essential component of cell membranes, where it plays a role in stabilizing transport across cell membranes and provides antioxidant protection.

Taurine plays a major role in good liver function via the formation of bile acids and detoxification. Abnormally low levels of taurine are common in many patients with chemical sensitivities and allergies. **Taurine is the major amino acid required by the liver for the removal of toxic chemicals and metabolites from the body**. Taurine is important for conjugation of drugs and metabolites in the liver via the acylation route. Once conjugated, chemical toxins are removed from the body as a component of bile and also through water soluble acetates in the urine. **Taurine is a key component of bile acids produced in the liver**. As bile synthesis utilizes cholesterol, disordered bile synthesis may result in elevated cholesterol.

Taurine is the body's main antioxidant defense against production of excess hypochlorite ion and if this is not controlled it will lead to severe aggravation of chemical sensitivity. Impaired body synthesis of taurine will reduce the ability of the liver to detoxify environmental chemicals such as chlorine, chlorite (bleach), aldehydes (produced from alcohol excess), alcohols, petroleum solvents, and ammonia. Taurine deficient persons are likely to have impaired mineral transport across the cell membrane, producing imbalances in electrolytes and reduced ability of the liver to remove pollutants via the excretory routes of the bowel and kidneys.

Recent findings are demonstrating that taurine is one of the major nutrients involved in the body's detoxification of harmful substances and drugs and should be considered in the treatment of all chemically sensitive patients. All good liver tonics should contain taurine.

Taurine is found in animal protein, organ meats, and invertebrate seafood and is often deficient in vegetarians. Factors that increase the body's requirements for taurine are vegetarianism, epilepsy, fad diets for rapid weight loss, alcohol, oral contraceptives, cortisone therapy, high stress levels, and a high intake of MSG.

Recommended dose of taurine is 200 to 500 mg daily.

Scientific reference: *Orthoplex Research Bulletin*, "Taurine the Detoxifying Amino Acid", Nutrients in Profile, by Henry Osiecki, Bioconcepts Publishing, Brisbane, Australia.

Dandelion

Dandelion is known by herbalists as *Taraxacum officinale* and its root has been used for liver and biliary complaints for centuries. Extensive records of its medicinal use exist from the tenth and eleventh centuries when it was promoted by famous Arabian doctors. In sixteenth-century Britain it was well established as an official drug of the apothecaries under the name of Herba Taraxacon and was a popular medicinal plant for the liver and digestive organs. Since the sixteenth century the Germans have used dandelion extensively for "blood purifying" and liver congestion. It is truly a universal herb and is still found in the official pharmacopeias of Switzerland, Poland, Hungary, and Russia. A huge amount of research has been carried out on the medicinal and nutritional effects of dandelion in many European countries. Dandelion has been used as a herbal medicine for centuries in China, India, and Nepal for liver ailments. Today dandelion is used widely as a liver tonic in North America, Australia, the Orient, and Europe.

The therapeutic properties of dandelion are due in part to its bitter substances taraxacin and inulin (a bitter glycoside). Other substances in dandelion are taraxanthin, sesquiterpenes, flavonoids, levulin, pectin, fatty acids, minerals, and vitamins.

Bitters, such as those in dandelion, stimulate the digestive glands and the liver and activate the flow of bile.

Although **dandelion's specific action is on the liver**, it also acts as a general body tonic. It acts as a laxative, diuretic, anti-inflammatory, bitter tonic, and cholagogue (a gallbladder tonic). Its cholagogue effect is useful for liver and gallbladder inflammation and congestion, as well as jaundiced states. It is of use in the early stages of cirrhosis of the liver, such as alcoholic cirrhosis.

Professor John King, the American doctor famous for his works on medicinal herbs, recommends dandelion for "weak digestion, loss of appetite, constipation, and hepatic (liver) torpor". Its dual liver and kidney action makes dandelion an excellent detoxifying remedy for gout, rheumatism, and skin complaints.

The *Australian Journal of Medical Herbalism*, Vol 3 (4), 1991, refers to two studies, which demonstrate the **liver healing properties of dandelion**. They found that dandelion successfully treats hepatitis, liver swelling, jaundice, and indigestion in those with inadequate bile secretion.

Dandelion leaves can be consumed fresh in salads, and dandelion root powder is a component of a liver tonic powder which is stirred into juices. The dried herb can be taken in capsule form. Doses range from 500 to 2000 mg daily. You can also buy dandelion tea and coffee or make your own beverage by adding one tablespoon of pieces of dried dandelion root to 16 fluid ounces of water in a saucepan, bring to a boil and simmer for 30 minutes. Strain and add honey to taste. This can be kept in the fridge and will give you a day's supply of refreshing beverage.

St Mary's Thistle (Milk Thistle)

This herb has been known as a **traditional liver tonic** for centuries and more than one hundred scientific research papers and a symposia have been produced on its liver-healing properties. Reference: *Australian Journal Medical Herbalism*, Vol 4 (1), 1992.; Lang I. et al, "Effect of the natural bioflavonoid anti-oxident silymarin on superoxide dismutase activity", *Biotechnol Ther:* 263-70, 1993.; Muzes G. et al."Effect of the bioflavonoid silymarin", *Acta Physiol Hung* 78: 3–9, 1991.; Valenzuela A. et al. "Selectivity of Silymarin", *Planta Med* 55: 420–22, 1989.; Carini R. et al. "Lipid preoxidation, protection by silybin", *Biochem Pharmacol* 43:2111–5, 1992.

Milk Thistle is also known as *Silybum marianum* or St. Mary's thistle.

Milk Thistle has **liver-protective, liver-regenerative**, anti-inflammatory, and antioxidant properties.

Milk Thistle can be used with benefit in the following conditions:

- chronic hepatitis
- cirrhosis
- liver damage
- bile stagnation (cholestasis)
- alcohol and chemical induced fatty liver

Clinical and laboratory studies and tissue examinations, both in humans and animals, have found Milk Thistle to have beneficial effects in treating all of the above.

Milk Thistle has been found to reduce toxic fatty degeneration of the liver.

In 1969 the renowned phalloidine experiment was carried out by the researchers Vogel and Temme (Reference: Arzneim Forsch 1969, 19:613-615). During this test, Milk Thistle was proven to be liver-protective. Phalloidine is extremely toxic to the liver. Milk Thistle can block its toxic effects, which indicates that it has powerful liver-protective capability.

Not only is this remarkable herb liver-protective, it has also been found to help liver cells (hepatocytes) repair and regenerate themselves after they have been damaged. Milk Thistle contains a flavone which protects some of the intracellular components of liver cells (mitochondria and microsomes) from lipid peroxidation; this protective effect upon the liver is much more powerful than that of vitamin E.

The powerful detoxification enzymes in the liver that break down drugs and toxic chemicals are called the cytochrome P450 enzymes. These enzymes are improved by one of the components of Milk Thistle called silibinin

A three-month study following sixty-seven patients with chronic hepatitis, toxic liver damage and biliary inflammation found that Milk Thistle greatly helped their liver disease. (Reference: S. Talalaj's research paper, *Silybum marianum*, Sydney, NHAA, 1985.) The same study found that patients with alcoholic cirrhosis had a significantly higher survival rate if treated with Milk Thistle.

Milk Thistle can be taken as capsules containing the dried herb or as a component of Livatone and Livatone Plus. Doses range from 500 to 2000mg daily.

Globe Artichoke

The herb globe artichoke, also known as *Cynara scolymus*, is a bitter tonic with **liver-protective and liver-restorative actions**. It has also been used as a "blood purifier". Clinical studies have established its value in lowering blood cholesterol, urea and nitrogen waste products of metabolism. (Reference: S. Rocchietta, Minerva Med 50,612, 1959.) It is of use as a liver restorative in cases of liver insufficiency and damage, liver diseases, poor digestion, gallstones, and chronic constipation. In overweight patients it can be used to lower elevated cholesterol and triglycerides. It can be used as a cleanser in cases of skin diseases, bad breath, and excessive body odor. Globe artichoke can be taken as capsules of the dried herb or as a component of Livatone powder which is stirred into juices. Doses range from 300 to 500 mg daily.

Slippery Elm Bark

The fine powder made from the bark of the slippery elm tree has a soothing effect upon the mucus membranes of the gastrointestinal tract. It produces temporary relief from the excessive acidity and reflux caused by digestive disorders. Slippery elm powder produces a protective lining upon inflamed and ulcerated mucosal surfaces and is thus of use for those with gastritis and stomach and duodenal ulcers. These types of gastro-intestinal problems are common in people with toxic livers and disordered bile production and slippery elm bark powder is most helpful in such cases, either mixed in juices by itself or as a component of a liver tonic powder. Doses range from 150 to 1000 mg daily but you can safely take more if needed.

HELPFUL FOODS FOR THE LIVER

The best vegetables for the liver are **carrots** and **beets** because they contain antioxidants such as beta-carotene, other carotenoids, and healing flavonoids which give color to these vegetables. These vegetable antioxidants have a healing and cleansing effect on the liver.

Lecithin helps the liver to metabolise fats and reduces high cholesterol levels. It also contains essential fatty acids and phosphatidylcholine which helps to keep the membranes around the liver cells (hepatocytes) healthy.

Alfalfa and **barley leaf** can be eaten to give your liver a boost of chlorophyll which is the green pigment that gives plants their color and enables them to convert solar energy into food energy. Chlorophyll acts as both a liver tonic and a liver cleanser.

HOW TO CHOOSE A GOOD LIVER TONIC

There are many liver tonics available today as medicine is finally starting to realize that common diseases such as obesity, chronic fatigue, digestive complaints, and allergies can be traced back to poor liver function. I personally do not think it is good to take liver tonics in the form of herbal tinctures containing alcohol, especially every day and on a long-term basis, as their alcohol content is not good for the liver. I prefer to use dried liver herbs mixed with peppermint leaf powder to give a pleasant and refreshing taste. There are some excellent liver tonic powders and capsules such as "LIVATONE" containing mixtures of psyllium, dandelion, Milk Thistle, globe artichoke, slippery elm bark, lecithin, barley leaf, carrot, beet powder, and alfalfa powder. They can be stirred into fresh juices and the natural peppermint herb gives a refreshing taste. All good liver tonics should contain the amino acid taurine, see page 66. A good quality liver tonic containing all the above ingredients is available under the brand of "Livatone". Livatone is available in capsule and powder form. For more information call 188875 LIVER

If you wish to order LivaTone you may do so by contacting S.C.B.

International at 1-888-782-7014 or Internet www.whas.com.au.

INTERESTING CASE HISTORIES

The Case of the Missing Gallstones

Juliette was typical of the women who gets gallstones, as doctors say, "fair, fat, and forty" and she came to see me initially as she felt unwell two years after her gallbladder was removed. This operation is called a cholecystectomy and Juliette's doctor had used the non-invasive method of removal using an operating telescope called a laparoscope, so that her scar was barely visible. Juliette was very disappointed as she had expected to feel much better and free of pain after her operation, especially as her surgeon had removed thirty-six small gallstones. However, she complained to me of abdominal bloating, constipation, heartburn, and weight gain of 55 pounds; no wonder she felt depressed!

Juliette's blood tests revealed an elevated cholesterol (262 mg/dl) and there was a slight elevation of her liver enzymes and bilirubin. My suspicions of poor liver function were confirmed by these blood tests and indeed her symptoms were typical of an overworked and tired liver. After the gallbladder is removed one needs to take extra care of the liver because the liver has to work harder at meal times without the gallbladder to provide stored bile at quick demand. I have also found that the condition of a fatty liver is more common after the gallbladder has been removed.

Juliette's dietary history revealed that she loved fatty foods such as cheese, chocolate, lamb chops, and packets of sweet cookies. Equally important was the lack of raw foods in her diet. She was in desperate need of the Liver-Cleansing Diet and was hugely relieved when I gave her this plan to follow as in the past she had been told to lose weight but had not been given a scientific method to follow. She was frightened of diets as she had a fear of hunger, so I spent some time telling her that she would never need to be hungry on the LCD as it was not about food restriction *per se*, it was simply a way of eating to restore metabolic balance and relieve her suffering.

Juliette returned after eight weeks having lost 25 pounds and said that her bloating had gone. Her cholesterol was down to 197 mg/dl and her liver function tests were completely normal. She told me that she wanted to stay on the LCD for another eight weeks and was ready to start it again as she wanted to lose more weight

Juliette told me a funny yet rather macabre story about how she lost her gallstones. Her surgeon had given her the thirty-six small hard stones containing bile acids and cholesterol to keep as a souvenir after her operation. On her return home from hospital she had the stones in a plastic bag and left them on her bedside table to show later to her husband Tom. Tom gave Juliette a special surprise and took her out that evening to a lovely movie to cheer her up after her illness. After returning home from the movie Juliette was sitting with Tom having a drink in the living room when they started to notice that there was a peculiar crunching sound emanating from the bedroom. After several minutes they became intrigued and wandered into the bedroom where, to their amazement, they discovered their pet dog Rufus merrily crunching away enjoying the last gallstone. Yes, Rufus had eaten all thirty-six gallstones depriving Juliette of her fascinating pathology specimen. Anyway, Rufus remained well and the gallstones appeared to have no adverse effects upon him. So the moral of this story is "don't leave your gallstones lying around if you want to keep them for posterity".

A HORMONAL CASE HISTORY

Ramona, aged twenty-six, came to see me because of a long-standing weight problem and hormonal imbalance. Those of you who know me may be aware that I have done a lot of research into the links between diet and body types and hormonal imbalances. If you would like to know more about this subject

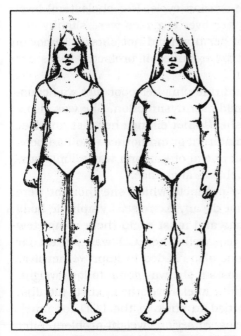

Lymphatic Shape (left) ideal weight, (right) overweight. See www.weightcontrol doctor.com Discover Your Body Type

I refer you to my book, *The Body Shaping Diet*, published in Australia by the Women's Health Advisory Service and by Time Warner in America.

Ramona was a typical "lymphatic" body type in that she was fat all over with a general thickness and puffiness in her limbs and body. Her ankles and wrists were puffy and swollen with fluid. She suffered with the allergies and excessive mucous production in her respiratory tract that is typical of lymphatic body types. She weighed 300 pounds and was so heavy that she had broken the bathroom scales at home. Her weight had gradually increased since adolescence when she had weighed around 154 pounds. She was a tall girl at 5 feet 10 inches but was still way too heavy for her frame (her body mass index was 45.7).

She complained that her menstrual periods had been absent for four years and she had headaches and sore breasts. I did blood tests and found that the level of the pituitary gland hormone called prolactin was too high which explained her lack of menstruation as high levels of prolactin switch off the ovarian cycle. Her cholesterol level was elevated at 278 mg/dl and her liver enzymes were slightly elevated. Thankfully, a CAT scan of her brain did not show a tumor of the pituitary gland which must be excluded if prolactin levels are high.

Ramona simply had obesity and this plus her poor diet was causing a hormonal imbalance and mild liver dysfunction. She was also a future candidate for diabetes if she did not change her diet and lose weight. She resembled her late maternal grandmother who had been very obese and diabetic. The task ahead of Ramona was a long journey of gradual weight loss and behavioral change.

Ramona was addicted to dairy products which she thought were good for her bones as she did not do any exercise. Lymphatic body types are allergic to dairy products and must avoid them completely if they are to lose weight and feel well. The LCD was perfect for Ramona as it is dairy free and she also needed to improve her liver function as shown by her blood tests if she was going to lose weight.

Ramona came to see me every four weeks over the next six months, as we had decided that she needed to stick to the LCD for much longer than eight weeks, because of her serious weight problem. After five months her blood tests for liver function were normal and her prolactin levels came down from 1500 to 350, heralded by the return of regular menstrual periods. The dairy-free diet had brought her prolactin down, cured her allergies and mucous problem, and made her feel much more energetic. Ramona was delighted and could not believe that she was as she said "melting away" so that she could see her bones reappearing underneath her previously swollen and puffy body. She told me that she had yearned for years to have bones like other girls so that she could wear dresses and skirts. By the end of the six months she had lost a whopping 105 pounds and weighed 195 pounds. She told me that now she felt human again, she was going to stay with the liver-cleansing foods and dairy-free diet forever.

It is very satisfying to help women like Ramona without drugs such as appetite suppressants or hormones, because, in the long term, these women do very well once they understand how to balance their metabolism and hormones through diet and exercise. Yes, the power of the LCD is enormous and can bring efficient and long-lasting weight loss for women and men with severe obesity whose future would otherwise be very bleak.

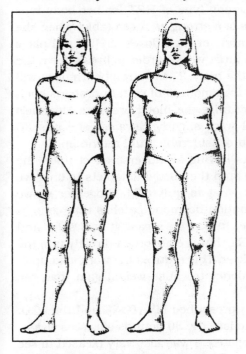

Android Shape (left) ideal weight, (right) overweight. See www.weightcontrol doctor.com Discover Your Body Type

A MENOPAUSAL CASE HISTORY

Now that all you post-war baby boomers, born in the late 1940s and 1950s are getting to menopause, I thought it appropriate to include a case history from a 54-year-old patient of mine called Joanne, I find a lot of women in the peri-menopausal age group are having problems controlling their weight.

Joanne was typical of my menopausal patients with weight problems who find that once they start taking hormone replacement therapy (HRT) their weight goes up and they start to feel sluggish. Joanne was an android body type meaning that she had a boyish figure with broad shoulders, strong shapely muscular arms and legs, narrow hips, a flat bottom, and not much of a waist. In android women the trunk is fairly straight up and down and the waist does not taper inwards. Weight gain tends to occur in the upper part of the body, especially around the waist so that a protuberant abdomen or "pot belly" occurs. Android women tend to be party animals and work their livers overtime with rich savory foods and alcohol. They love cheeses, hams, anchovies, chips and fried foods and Joanne had all these characteristics. I have found that many overweight android- shaped people have a fatty liver. The incidence of fatty liver is much greater in android-shaped people and may be associated with high blood fats and cardiovascular disease.

Joanne had been given the wrong type of HRT for her body type and was taking fairly high doses of a strong estrogen tablet when she first came to see me. Strong brands or high doses of HRT will place extra burden on the liver which must work harder to break down the hormones for elimination from the body. These strong hormones will also induce the liver to make extra amounts of certain proteins such as clotting factors and this may raise the blood pressure. Joanne's blood pressure and cholesterol were slightly elevated, she was 30 pounds overweight, and she had considerable fluid retention.

I explained that her HRT was having an adverse effect upon the liver and that we would have to stop the hormone tablets to improve her liver function. She did not want to quit HRT altogether so we switched her to the new combination hormone patches that contain both estrogen and progesterone. In Joanne's case it was safer and more natural to give forms of HRT that are absorbed directly into the circulation, thus bypassing the liver. This reduces the work load upon the liver and will have less tendency to cause weight gain than the tablet (oral) forms of HRT.

To help Joanne's weight loss I prescribed LIVATONE and the LCD. It took four months for Joanne to lose the 30 pounds of excess weight that she had gained since menopause. I was also very pleased to see her blood pressure and cholesterol had come down nicely with the balancing effect of the LCD. If you wish to discuss the use of hormone patches and creams, or liver tonics you may talk to your own doctor or visit us on the Internet at www.liverdoctor.com or write to Dr. Cabot at PO Box 5070 Glendale AZ 85312 - 5070.

Chapter 7

THE PHILOSOPHY OF THE LIVER-CLEANSING DIET

Before we launch ourselves into the delicious and cleansing meal plans and recipes of the Liver-Cleansing Diet (LCD) I am going to give you an outline of the philosophy and logistics of the diet. The LCD is based on my many years of experience in treating diseases with nutritional medicine and has been proven to work time and time again, often in cases where conventional medicine had very little to offer the patient. I have successfully used this diet to restore health in patients with such diverse health problems as obesity, alcoholic liver damage, immune dysfunction such as severe allergies and auto-immune diseases, headaches, chronic fatigue, depression, skin diseases, arthritis, chronic constipation, irritable bowel syndrome, ulcerative colitis, Crohn's disease, recurrent bowel infections, candida, and excessive exposure to toxins such as insecticides and drugs. Furthermore, the LCD can often rejuvenate those with generally poor health of unknown cause which is very important as many of these patients struggle through life feeling tired and irritable—which is harder to bear if you cannot find a cause and thus see no prospect of relief.

A healthy liver keeps the body clean, thereby protecting the immune system from overload and is fundamental to efficient metabolism and body weight control. Poor liver function, even of a slight degree, can cause far reaching and diverse health problems, such as those described above. By improving liver function through diet and various liver tonics these multiple and sometimes seemingly unrelated health problems will be alleviated or at the least greatly reduced.

My LCD will enable you to lose weight and feel more energetic, even if all other diets have let you down and your life has been one long "yo-yo" journey to ever-increasing weight. This time it

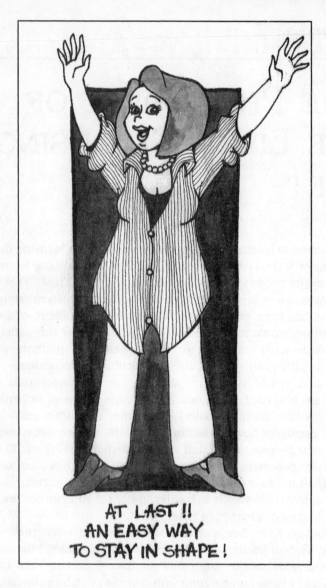

AT LAST !!
AN EASY WAY
TO STAY IN SHAPE !

will be different, I can assure you. The LCD will make you slim
and healthy.

The LCD will work for you, and anyone with a weight problem,
and it is the only scientific eating plan ever devised by a doctor
to improve liver function. In the first part of this book I have
shown you that the liver is the supreme organ of metabolism and

is the only body organ that can pump fat out of the body. The key to successful weight loss and maintenance is to restore efficient liver function which is not hard to do when you have the information in this book.

I do hope that the case histories from several of my patients who have followed the LCD and found excellent results (see pages 72 to 76) have given you inspiration. For ethical reasons the names of the patients have been changed, but the details of these case histories are true and factual. Some sound too good to be true and I must admit that in the early days of prescribing the LCD I was often amazed at the good results my patients were obtaining from the diet. Some of these patients would find my amazement amusing and some kindly offered to be a guest on my radio show to tell others of their success. After the show we would always have hundreds of inquiries which prompted me to put the LCD into a proper book.

Thus you can begin the LCD with great enthusiasm and confidence and I would like to hear from you at the end of eight weeks to learn of your success. Email Dr Sandra Cabot, at usahelp@qwest.net.

LET'S TALK ABOUT FOOD

You will enjoy the food in the LCD as the recipes are light, nutritionally balanced and flavorful. I have worked with several women who are excellent cooks to bring you the culinary delights found in the LCD. The wonderful women who have helped me make the LCD a delicious journey are Wendy Mawson (a superb cook), Beverley Clarke, a body-shaping counselor, my sister Madeleine McRae, Florence Thomas, and Kaye Tonkin—as they say, variety is the spice of life, and on the LCD you definitely won't get bored.

The LCD is very simple which makes it easy to follow and increases your chance of success. There is no need to remember complex food combining rules or to painstakingly count every calorie or gram of fat. You just need to relax and follow the menus given for the eight weeks that you will be on this diet.

If you are away, or can't find this book, or don't have time to cook, it is still possible to stay on the LCD by sticking to its twelve vital principles on pages 45 to 65, until you can return to normal.

If for some reason you blow it and go on a twenty-four-hour cheese and chocolate binge or have a few too many drinks, don't despair! All you need do is return to the LCD and add two extra days to the eight weeks. I can hear you saying, "Why two extra days when I only blew it for one day?" The answer is that if you overload your liver with fat, sugar, or alcohol while you are in the middle of the Liver-Cleansing Diet you create greater metabolic disturbance than if you did it while you are eating and drinking in the "average" manner typical of affluent societies.

Chapter 8

THE EIGHT-WEEK EATING PLAN

The LCD is an **eight-week eating plan** that gives you plenty of variety and well-balanced and nutritious meals. You will need to stay on it for eight weeks to fully cleanse and rejuvenate your liver; however, you can safely stay on it for much longer if you find that you have more weight to lose at the end of the eight weeks. The average weight loss over the eight-week period is 22 pounds, but in some people it can be much more. I have found that a good liver tonic (see page 71) can increase the amount of weight loss because of its effect in improving liver function. Some people return to the Liver-Cleansing Diet again and again to maintain a healthy body weight and also because they feel so much better when they are on it. It is quite safe and beneficial to stay on the LCD indefinitely, especially if you have liver disease or problems with your immune system. There are plenty of recipes and healthy eating suggestions so that you can vary the menus quite a lot.

After you have finished the eight-week eating plan, I suggest that you continue to eat in a "liver-conscious" way by staying within the basic guidelines and following the twelve vital liver-cleansing principles found on pages 45 to 65. This will keep your weight under control and your general energy levels high. If your weight begins to creep up, you are probably eating too much fat and I suggest you return to the LCD for another eight weeks.

The LCD is a great way of eating for both men and women, and many men who enjoy a few drinks find it an excellent way to keep their liver in tip-top shape.

If you suffer with **any** serious or chronic medical problems such as diabetes, blood clots or kidney disease, you should only follow the LCD under the supervision of your own doctor. The LCD has not been designed for pregnant or breast-feeding women, who have special nutritional needs; they must take the advice of their own doctor or dietician.

The first two weeks of the LCD are fairly gentle and not rigorous because the liver may have a high level of toxins and accumulated fatty substances and we do not want to release these into your circulation too quickly as this can cause an unpleasant elimination reaction.

The middle four weeks of the LCD are more demanding because by this time both you and your liver will be accustomed to a low-fat diet and you will be feeling more energetic. Hang in there during these four weeks as it is necessary to really cleanse the liver if we are to stimulate your sluggish metabolism and speed up weight loss. If you feel a little tired or have a few headaches, please **drink extra water** to flush those toxins out of the body during this critical time.

The last two weeks of the LCD are less demanding than the middle four weeks, but they are more demanding than the first two weeks. This is because you need to make a smooth transition back to your general way of eating once you have finished the LCD.

Once again I do recommend that you stick to the twelve strategies for liver health on pages 45 to 65 once you have finished the eight-week LCD as you will want to maintain a dynamic metabolism by keeping your liver healthy.

On the LCD you will eat a lot of raw fruits and vegetables as these are what your liver craves. Raw foods are liver-cleansing and around 40 percent of your diet will consist of raw vegetables and fruits. In particular, dark green leafy vegetables and orange and red-colored fruits and vegetables contain living enzymes, natural antibiotics, chlorophyll, carotenoids, and bioflavonoids that will heal your liver and cleanse the bowel.

Raw vegetables and fruits will reduce excess acidity, thereby making your body's biochemical acid-base balance more alkaline and this is most important for those with excessive inflammation.

Most people do not eat sufficient raw vegetables and fruits and the LCD will inspire you to do this as the salad recipes are delicious and we teach you how to prepare these foods in an appetizing way. There are lovely salad dressings that will make you a salad lover forever!

Sources of protein for the LCD are legumes, grains, seeds, and nuts in various combinations, fish and seafood, as well as free-range chicken and eggs. No other meats or dairy products should be eaten on the LCD.

Although I do not include red meats, pork, or fowl (other than some free-range chicken) in the Liver-Cleansing Diet I do not think that these foods are unhealthy if eaten in moderation (say three to four times a week). When and if you do eat these meats always use low-fat varieties, trim off all the fat, and do not fry or bake them in fat.

During the middle four weeks there are more vegetarian meals and no chicken or egg yolks are allowed.

Breakfast is generally light and consists of raw fruits, and cereals with soy, rice, or almond milks.

For those who love breakfast or those who expend a lot of physical energy during the morning, we have been very creative and have delicious fruit smoothies, pancakes, savory jaffles (toasted sandwiches), soy-bean burgers, and home-made muffins to choose from.

If you have liver disease or feel that your metabolism is very sluggish you can confine yourself to raw fruits and raw juices for breakfast as this is the most cleansing program of all. This is similar in principle to the "fit for life" diet where only raw foods are eaten up until lunch time.

However, the LCD gives you the option of more variety for breakfast, especially for people who may need to do physical labor in the mornings. For those who suffer with low blood sugar (hypoglycemia) in the mid-morning it is often necessary to choose one of the more substantial breakfast menus which contains protein as well as some raw fruit. By having some protein for breakfast your blood sugar levels will be more stable.

If you want to lose weight at a faster pace, or if you have a lot of weight to lose, say more than 44 pounds, then the option of confining breakfast to just raw fruits and juices will be more effective. Many people really enjoy following the LCD because it gives them so many choices and they can tailor-make a dietary program within its menus to suit their individual requirements.

Lunch and Dinner recipes can be interchangeable so that if you feel like a large lunch you may use a dinner recipe and then use the lighter lunch recipe for dinner. If you feel like a substantial meal have a soup and main course **or** a main course followed by a dessert. **On the LCD you should not have more than two courses in any one**

meal as poor or excessive food combining places a heavy work load upon the liver.

There are a great variety of main courses and soups to choose from and if you are not very hungry I suggest you choose a lighter alternative such as a salad, a salad sandwich, or just one of our delicious liver-cleansing soups. Remember, liver strategy number one is to listen to your body (see page 45). If you are not hungry at all when lunch or dinner time arrives, just have a salad or a juice as your liver may be working hard to eliminate all those accumulated fats and toxins from years of eating poorly. This is sacred work so don't interrupt it. Remember, it is acceptable to miss meals if you are not hungry and that animals who are underfed live longer. Don't feel guilty if you miss a meal, just have a juice or piece of fruit or a salad instead. Fasting has been used since time immemorial as an aid to rejuvenation.

Desserts or sweets are provided for on the LCD as some people must have something sweet to finish off their evening meal. We have simple fruit salad sweets and also some very exotic and even "naughty" sweet treats on the LCD. Of course, they are not *really* naughty as we cannot give you sweets that would stop the process of liver-cleansing.

If you feel full after eating your main course I suggest you only have raw fruit for dessert, or skip it altogether. Remember to listen to your real hunger and not your mind's hunger.

Snacks between meals are fine if you become hungry. On the LCD you can have a maximum of three main meals daily with small snacks in between, although I suggest you do not have more than two or three snacks daily, especially if trying to lose weight.

Snacks may consist of raw carrot and celery sticks, one orange, one apple or a handful of raw almonds, raw cashews, seeds, and raisins. Another snack that you can have is one rice cake spread with avocado or hummus.

Instead of eating a snack why not have a raw juice? Try carrot, celery, beet, apple, spinach, and fresh ginger root in various combinations. You will need a good quality juice extracting machine while on the LCD as raw juices are powerful healing and cleansing tonics for the liver. **Raw juices make the best snacks of all for those on the LCD.** *If you have a sensitive stomach or want to increase fluid intake, dilute the juices with filtered water and/or ice cubes.*

Remember that **certain snacks are not liver-cleansing** and we suggest you avoid them. Snacks to avoid are: all dairy products e.g.

dairy milk, butter, cheese, cream, yogurt, ice cream, chocolate, chips, French fries, salted pretzels, salted or roasted nuts, preserved meats, sweet cookies and cakes, candies, ice creams, and anything that is found in a packet and loaded with chemicals, salt and damaged fats. These things will give your liver a beating.

BASIC MENU PLAN

The menus in the LCD are simple and easy to follow. They are divided into three sections:

1. **SECTION ONE—The first two weeks:**
   Menus are found on pages 86 to 92. There are many different breakfasts, lunches, and dinners to choose from so you have plenty of variety. The page references for all recipes are given and all recipes appear in the back section of the book.

2. **SECTION TWO—The middle four weeks:**
   Menus are found on pages 92 to 99. There are many different breakfasts, lunches, and dinners to choose from so you have plenty of variety. The page references for all recipes are given and all recipes appear in the back section of the book.

3. **SECTION THREE—The last two weeks:**
   Menus are found on pages 99 to 105. There are many different breakfasts, lunches, and dinners to choose from so you have plenty of variety. The page references for all recipes are given and all recipes appear in the back section of the book.

You do not have to try all the recipes and if there are some that don't appeal, you may omit them. If there are recipes that you adore or make you feel terrific you may repeat them within the appropriate section of the diet. Remember that it is important to stick to the menus within each section while you are still on that particular section. In other words, don't go eating recipes from section one (the first two weeks) while you are in section two (the middle four weeks) or you will slow down the liver-cleansing process.

MENU PLANS FOR LIVER-CLEANSING DIET

SECTION ONE—THE FIRST TWO WEEKS

BREAKFASTS—SECTION ONE

First thing on arising drink 2 large glasses of purified water with the juice of a fresh lemon, lime, or orange to cleanse the liver. Fifteen minutes later have a raw vegetable juice made with carrot, celery, and parsley.

You may have any of the following:

1. Fresh fruit salad using any seasonal fruits. You may add 3–4 tablespoons LSA (page 146) as this will give you protein and extra fiber. You may also add 4–5 tablespoons Fruit and Nut Cream (page 146) to the fruit salad if desired.

2. 2 Whole wheat Pancakes (page 151) which may be topped with fresh fruits, lemon, or orange juice with honey, chopped nuts, and some LSA mixture.

3. Rusher's Shake (page 144) is great if you want a quick, light, and easily digested breakfast.

4. Cereals such as unsweetened or home-made muesli, Special K, or cooked rolled oats. Use around 1½ ounces cereal. Use soy, almond, or rice milk. You may add fresh banana, apple, or apricots to the cereal if desired and 3–4 tablespoons LSA for extra protein.

5. Toast—2–3 slices using whole wheat, buckwheat, sour dough rye, or other high-quality bread from the health food store. You may have a sweet topping such as tahini, honey, and LSA; banana, honey, and LSA, or our own Apricot Jelly (page 146). You can also use our Pineapple Ginger Spread (page 146) or

mashed banana with blueberries and lemon juice, or sliced banana topped with kiwifruit and sprinkled with LSA. Please avoid jellies, jams, and commercial preserves.

If you prefer you may have a savory topping on your toast such as boiled, poached or curried free-range eggs (page 151) or Grilled Tomatoes (page 152), or sardines, salmon, tuna, or fresh Cooked Mushrooms (page 152). Another nice topping for toast is freshly sliced avocado with a squeeze of lime or lemon juice, finely chopped scallions, and black pepper. Our yummy Tofu Spread (page 147) is also nice on toast.

6. Muffins—banana and walnut or apple flavored (page 148 and 149). I suggest you have 1–2 pieces fresh fruit with 1–2 muffins.

7. 1 bowl cooked brown rice (around 2½ ounces) with wheatgerm and 3 tablespoons LSA. Add soy milk and fresh fruit, such as bananas and strawberries, or raisins.

8. Jaffles (toasted sandwiches) (page 151) with a savory filling are great in winter. You may have a raw vegetable salad, such as lettuce, cherry tomatoes, and carrots on the side.

9. Soya Bean Burger (page 149) with a side salad of cucumber, cherry tomatoes, and carrots.

10. Scrambled Tofu (page 152) with a side salad of cherry tomatoes, carrot sticks, and sliced apple.

LUNCHES—SECTION ONE

You may have any of the following:

1. Sandwiches using whole wheat bread, sour dough rye bread, stone ground bread, rice bread, corn bread, herb and olive bread, walnut bread, or any high-quality bread from the health food store. You may spread the bread with avocado, tahini, or Hummus (page 147). Do not use any butter or margarine.
    For sandwich fillings use finely grated raw carrot, raw zuc-

chini, raw beet, and raw winter squash. You may add canned fish such as sardines, tuna, or red or pink salmon if desired.

Another healthy and tasty sandwich filling is Tofu Spread (page 147).

Other suggested fillings are tofu with grated carrot and golden raisins; tuna with grated carrot, lettuce, and red onion rings; strips of free-range chicken, tomato, onion, lettuce, and chopped fresh mint; sliced free-range hard-boiled eggs with lettuce and cucumber; sliced avocado with steamed broccoli and a dash of balsamic vinegar or salt-reduced soy sauce; tahini, grated carrot, and dried apricots.

To add flavor to sandwiches you may use freshly ground black pepper or lemon pepper, chopped coriander/cilantro, chives or scallions/green onions.

2. Avocado, Orange, and Mushroom Salad (page 119). You may have 1–2 slices of bread with this, plus 1 free-range hard-boiled egg or 3 ounces canned tuna.

3. Spicy Seafood Salad (page 123) with a side salad of grated carrot, beet, cherry tomatoes, and cucumber.

4. Tuna and Pasta Salad (page 128).

5. Apple, Carrot, and Beet Salad (page 132) with ½ breast or 1 drumstick of free-range skinless chicken.

6. Melon and Chicken Breast Salad (page 131).

7. Potato and Leek Soup (page 134) with 1 slice of toast spread with mashed avocado and sprinkled with LSA, and a small side salad of celery, tomato, and sliced apple.

8. Pumpkin Soup (page 140) with 1 slice of toast spread with tahini, and topped with chopped coriander/cilantro, chives, and parsley.

9. Chicken Soup à la Madeleine (page 141) garnished with a side salad of lettuce, celery, bell pepper, and sliced carrots.

10. Leek and Lentil Soup à la Florentine (page 137) with 1 slice of

toast spread with Hummus (page 147), and topped with grated raw carrot, beet and zucchini. Flavor with freshly ground black pepper and chives if desired.

11. Mixed Bean Salad (page 124) with a side salad of grated carrot and beet, cherry tomatoes, bell pepper, and lettuce sprinkled with LSA.

12. Pita Pizza (page 168) with a side salad of lettuce, grated raw carrot and beet, bell pepper, and cucumber.

13. Terrific Tuna, Tomatoes, and Pasta (page 169) with a side salad of lettuce, grated raw carrot and beet, bell pepper and cucumber.

14. Savory Crepes (page 155) with a side salad of parsley, cherry tomatoes, carrot sticks, lettuce, and bell pepper.

16. Carrot Sunflower Seed Surprise (page 156).

17. Zucchini and Herb Omelette (page 154) with a side salad of parsley, cherry tomatoes, carrot sticks, lettuce, and bell pepper.

18. Wild Rice and Creamed Spinach (page 176) with a side salad of lettuce, tomatoes, and cucumber.

19. Dolmades, which are stuffed vine leaves (page 155), with a side salad of parsley, cherry tomatoes, carrot sticks, lettuce, and bell pepper.

20. Spaghetti with Chili Tomato Sauce (page 160) with a side salad of grated raw beet, carrot and zucchini, parsley, and scallions/green onions.

21. Red Lentils with Artichokes (page 167) sprinkled with LSA and garnished with a side salad of grated raw beet, carrot, zucchini, parsley, and scallions/green onions.

22. You may have any one of our yummy salads (pages 119 to 132) and salad dressings (pages 114 to 118), with 2 slices of toast, or 2 crackers, or rice cakes.

EVENING MEAL—SECTION ONE

You may have any soup (see soup recipes pages 133 to 143) **or** any dessert (see dessert recipes pages 178 to 186) with any of the following main courses. Do not have more than 2 courses for the evening meal (i.e. don't have a soup and main course and dessert which would be 3 courses as this will overwork the liver and slow down digestion and metabolism). **Always have a raw vegetable salad with your main course as this will improve digestion**. You may have a light salad dressing if desired. If you have a weak digestive system try slowly sipping 1 small glass of water containing 1 teaspoon of non-alcoholic apple cider vinegar during the meal.

If you don't have much of an appetite for dinner, skip the main course altogether and just have soup and toast or one of our lovely salads (see salad recipes pages 119 to 132).

For chicken dishes use only free-range skinless chicken.

You may have any of the following:

1. Vegetable Ratatouille (page 171) with 1 bowl brown rice sprinkled with LSA.

2. Steamed Fish with Ginger and Scallions (page 170).

3. Stuffed Bell Peppers (page 171).

4. Kay Bell's Chicken Paradiso (page 173).

5. Fried Rice with Egg and Vegetables (page 177).

6. Bakmi Goreng (page 173). This is nice if you like Indonesian food.

7. Wild Rice Stuffed Tomatoes (page 153) with 2 baked potatoes.

8. Herbed, Steamed Fish Fillets (page 154).

9. Wild Mushroom and Chestnut Ragout (page 175).

10. Spicy Chicken Kebabs (page 157).

11.   Zucchini and Herb Omelette (page 154).

12.   Vegetable Casserole (page 156).

13.   Chicken and Almonds (page 169).

14.   Stuffed Potatoes with Baked Beans (page 157).

15.   Grilled Fish of choice and Winter Squash Baked with Sesame Seeds (page 158).

16.   Chicken Chow Mein (page 159).

17.   Spaghetti with Chili Tomato Sauce (page 160).

18.   Family Fish Cakes (page 161).

19.   Hot Vegetable Curry (page 163).

20.   Easy Chicken and Leek Casserole (page 162).

21.   Beans with Mushrooms (page 163).

22.   Fried Rice with Shrimp (page 164).

23.   Golden Casserole (page 165).

24.   Spicy Chicken Sauce and Pasta (page 166).

25.   Ratatouille Kebabs (page 167).

26.   Grilled Ocean Perch (Orange Roughy) with Fennel (page 169).

27.   Whole Fish Chinese Style (page 158).

28.   Salmon and Basil Loaf (page 168).

29.   Wild Rice and Creamed Spinach (page 176).

SECTION TWO—THE MIDDLE FOUR WEEKS

BREAKFASTS—SECTION TWO

First thing on arising drink 2 large glasses of purified water with the juice of a fresh lemon, lime, or orange to cleanse the liver. Fifteen minutes later have a raw vegetable juice made with carrot, celery, and parsley.

You may have any of the following:

1. Fresh fruit salad using 3–4 pieces of seasonal fruit. You may add 2–4 tablespoons LSA (page 146) for extra protein and fiber or our Fruit and Nut Cream (page 146).

2. Raw vegetable and/or fruit juice made with a juice extracting machine. Good combinations are carrot, beet, celery, apple, pear, orange, and ginger. Be adventurous and try different combinations of these. You may dilute with water or ice cubes if desired.

3. Toast—2–3 slices using whole wheat, buckwheat, sour dough rye, or other high-quality bread from the health food store. You may have a sweet topping such as tahini, honey, and LSA; banana, honey, and LSA, or our own Apricot Jelly (page 146) or Pineapple Ginger Spread (page 146). Toast may be topped with mashed banana with blueberries and lemon juice, or sliced banana and kiwifruit sprinkled with LSA. Please avoid jams, jellies, and commercial preserves.

   If you prefer you may have a savory topping on your toast such as Grilled Tomatoes (page 152), or sardines, salmon, tuna, or fresh Cooked Mushrooms (page 152). Another nice topping for toast is freshly sliced avocado with a squeeze of lime or lemon juice, finely chopped scallions, and freshly ground black pepper. Our yummy Tofu Spread (page 147) is also nice on toast.

   Note that during Section Two egg yolks should be avoided.

4. 1 bowl cooked brown rice (around 2½ ounces) with 1 tablespoon wheatgerm and 3 tablespoons LSA. Add soy milk and fresh fruit,

such as bananas and strawberries, or raisins, prunes, or dried apricots. You may also add our delicious Fruit and Nut Cream (page 146).

5.   Cereals such as unsweetened or home-made muesli, Special K, or cooked rolled oats. Use around 1½ ounces cereal. Use soy, almond, or rice milk. You may add 3–4 tablespoons LSA for extra protein. You may add fresh banana, apple, or apricots to the cereal if desired.

6.   Easy Fruit Shake. Place ½ cup unsweetened canned pears, apricots, or peaches in a blender with 4 fluid ounces soy or rice milk, 1 tablespoon lecithin granules, 2 tablespoons LSA, and 1 teaspoon wheatgerm. Blend together until smooth and add ice cubes if desired.

7.   Golden Fruit Salad made with sliced papaya, cantaloupe, peach (canned peaches in natural juice may be substituted), and mango with freshly squeezed orange juice. Sprinkle 2 tablespoons LSA on top.

8.   Rusher's Shake (page 144) is great if you want a light, quick, and easily digested breakfast.

9.   Nanastrawki Shake (page145) is a high energy and filling liquid breakfast.

10.   Melon Magic Health Shake (page144) is a very light and refreshing liquid breakfast.

11.   Summer Punch (page 144) is very light and cleansing and great for weight watchers.

12.   Rice cakes with Hummus (page 147), sliced tomato, parsley, and Avocado Spread (page 147).

13.   Soup of Fruit (page 139) is a nice exotic chilled soup on a hot summer morning. Your liver-conscious friends will like this for brunch. Serve it with slices of fresh fruit on the side.

14. Scrambled Tofu (page 152) with a side salad of cherry tomatoes, carrot sticks, and sliced apple.

LUNCHES—SECTION TWO

You may have any of the following:

1. Wild Rice and Creamed Spinach (page 176) with a side salad of lettuce, tomatoes, and cucumber.

2. Red Lentils with Artichokes (page 167) sprinkled with LSA and garnished with a side salad of grated raw beet, carrot, and zucchini, parsley, and scallions/green onions.

3. Terrific Tuna, Tomatoes, and Pasta (page 169) with a side salad of lettuce, grated raw carrot and beet, bell pepper and cucumber.

4. Leek and Lentil Soup à la Florentine (page 137) with 1 slice toast spread with Hummus (page 147) and topped with grated raw carrot, beet and zucchini. Flavor with freshly ground black pepper and chives if desired.

5. Sprout Salad (page 122) with one of our salad dressings and add 3–5 ounces canned red salmon on the side.

6. Bamboo Shoot, Carrot, and Raisin Salad (page 122) with one of our dressings and Tabbouleh (page 125). Sprinkle with LSA.

7. Avocado, Mango, and Lime Salad (page 126) with Corn and Rice Delight (page 127).

8. Crustacean Salad (page 128) with 3 celery sticks.

9. Mixed Bean Salad (page 124) with a side salad of grated carrot and beet, cherry tomatoes, bell pepper, and lettuce sprinkled with LSA.

10. Potato and Vegetable Salad (page 129) with rice cakes spread

with Hummus (page 147) and chopped chives or scallions/green onions and sprinkled with LSA.

11. Asparagus Spears and Lettuce Salad (page 130) and 1–2 slices whole wheat or sour dough rye bread topped with Tofu Spread (page 147).

12. Rice Harvest Salad (page 127) and Garden Fresh Green Salad (page 126).

13. Pasta Salad with Avocado (page 131) and Zucchini Salad (page 130).

14. Apple, Carrot, and Beet Salad (page 132) with 1–2 slices toast topped with sardines and scallions/green onions.

15. Snow Pea Salad (page 132) with Minestrone Soup (page 142) and 1 slice dry toast.

16. Potato and Leek Soup (page 134) with 2 slices toast topped with Hummus (page 147), grated raw carrot and beet and sprinkled with LSA.

17. Haricot (or Navy) Bean Soup (page 133) with 1 small bowl brown rice, 1 teaspoon cold-pressed virgin olive oil (if desired), chopped chives, and dried tomatoes. Season with freshly ground black pepper if desired.

18. Sandwiches using whole wheat bread, sour dough rye bread, stone ground bread, rice bread, corn bread, herb and olive bread, walnut bread, or any high-quality bread from the health food store. You may spread the bread with avocado, tahini, or Hummus (page 147). Do not use any butter or margarine.

    For sandwich fillings use finely grated raw carrot, raw zucchini, raw beet and raw winter squash, and you may add canned fish, such as sardines, tuna, or red or pink salmon if desired.

    Another healthy and tasty sandwich filling is Tofu Spread (page 147).

    Other suggested sandwich fillings are tofu with grated carrot and golden raisins, tuna with grated carrot, lettuce and red onion rings; tomato, onion, lettuce, and chopped fresh mint; sliced avocado with steamed broccoli and a dash of balsamic vinegar or salt-reduced soy sauce; tahini, grated carrot, and dried apricots.

To add flavor to sandwiches you may add freshly ground black pepper or lemon pepper, chopped coriander/cilantro, chives or scallions/green onions.

19. Wild Rice Stuffed Tomatoes (page 153) with a side salad of grated raw carrots and beets, sunflower seeds, cucumber, parsley, and dressing of choice.

20. Noodle Soup (page 133) with 2 rice cakes topped with tahini, sliced tomatoes, parsley, sliced cucumber and LSA.

21. Split Pea Soup (page 138) with 2 slices toast topped with baked beans, chives, and parsley.

22. Mushroom Consommé (page 140) with 2 rice cakes topped with tuna or red salmon, lettuce, and parsley.

23. Pasta Salad with Avocado, (page 131) and Coleslaw (page 130) sprinkled with LSA.

24. Tuna and Pasta Salad (page 128).

25. Cherry Tomato, Avocado and Grapefruit Salad (page 128) and Grilled Ocean Perch (Orange Roughy) with Fennel (page 169).

26. Spicy Shrimp with Brussels Sprouts (page 161) with a side salad of grated raw carrot and beet and parsley.

27. Buckwheat and Vegetables (page 172) sprinkled with LSA and garnished with a side salad of carrot sticks, celery sticks, apple and walnuts.

28. Mushrooms with Walnuts and Walnut Oil Dressing (page 125) and fresh garden salad with sunflower seeds and 1 small bowl brown rice.

29.   Tabbouleh (page 125) with 2 rice cakes topped with Tofu Spread (page 147).

30.   Whole wheat pasta with a selection of vegetables stir-fried with garlic, onions, reduced-salt soy sauce or tomato paste, freshly ground black pepper, and chili (optional). Sprinkle with LSA.

EVENING MEALS—SECTION TWO

You may have any soup (see soup recipes pages 133 to 143) **or** any dessert (see dessert recipes pages 178 to 186) with any of the following main courses. Do not have more than 2 courses for the evening meal (i.e. don't have a soup and main course and dessert which would be 3 courses as this will overwork the liver and slow down digestion and metabolism). Always have a raw vegetable salad with your main course as this will improve digestion. You may have a light salad dressing if desired. If you have a weak digestive system try slowly sipping 1 small glass of water containing 1 teaspoon apple cider vinegar during the meal.

If you don't have much of an appetite for dinner, skip the main course altogether and just have soup and toast or one of our lovely salads (see recipes for salads page 119 to 132).

During the middle four weeks (section two) you need to avoid chicken and egg yolks, however seafood is allowed. In the recipes where a choice of chicken stock or vegetable stock is given, use vegetable stock.

You may have any of the following:

1.   Wild Rice Stuffed Tomatoes (page 153).

2.   Herbed, Steamed Fish Fillets (page 154).

3.   Wild Mushroom and Chestnut Ragout (page 175).

4.   Vegetable Casserole (page 156) with 1 bowl brown rice sprinkled with LSA.

5.   Stuffed Potatoes with Baked Beans (page 157).

6.   Winter Squash Baked with Sesame Seeds (page 158) and grilled fish of choice.

7.   Whole Fish Chinese Style (page 158).

8.   Soya Bean Burgers (page 159).

9.   Spaghetti with Chili Tomato Sauce (page 160).

10.   Family Fish Cakes (page 161).

11.   Hot Vegetable Curry (page 163).

12.   Beans with Mushrooms (page 163).

13.   Fried Rice with Shrimp (page 164).

14.   Golden Casserole (page 165).

15.   Spicy Shrimp with Brussels Sprouts (page 161).

16.   Scallops with Crushed Sesame Seeds (page 164).

17.   Red Lentils with Artichokes (page 167) with 1 bowl brown rice sprinkled with LSA.

18.   Ratatouille Kebabs (page 167) with 1 bowl brown rice sprinkled with LSA.

19.   Pita Pizza (page 168).

20.   Grilled Salmon Cutlets (page 166).

21.   Grilled Ocean Perch (Orange Roughy) with Fennel (page 169).

22.   Terrific Tuna, Tomatoes, and Pasta (page 169).

23.   Vegetable Ratatouille (page 171).

24.   Steamed Fish with Ginger and Scallions (page 170).

SECTION THREE—THE LAST TWO WEEKS

BREAKFASTS—SECTION THREE

First thing on arising drink 2 large glasses of purified water with the juice of a fresh lemon, lime, or orange to cleanse the liver. Fifteen minutes later have a raw vegetable juice made with carrot, celery, and parsley.

You may have any of the following:

1.   Toast—2–3 slices using whole wheat, buckwheat, sour dough rye, or other high-quality bread from the health food store. You may have a sweet topping such as tahini, honey, and LSA; banana, honey, and LSA, or our own Apricot Jelly (page 146) or Pineapple Ginger Spread (page 146). You may also top your toast with mashed banana, blueberries, and lemon juice, or sliced banana and kiwifruit sprinkled with LSA. Please avoid jams, jellies, and commercial preserves.

   If you prefer you may have a savory topping on your toast such as free-range eggs (boiled, poached or curried (see egg recipes page 151) or Grilled Tomatoes (page 152), or sardines, salmon, tuna, or fresh Cooked Mushrooms (page 152). Another nice topping for toast is freshly sliced avocado with a squeeze of lime or lemon juice, finely chopped scallions/green onions, and freshly ground black pepper. Our yummy Tofu Spread (page 147) is also nice on toast.

2. Cereals such as unsweetened or home-made muesli, Special K, cooked rolled oats. Use around 1½ ounces cereal. Use soy, almond, or rice milk. You may add 3–4 tablespoons LSA for extra protein. You may also add fresh banana, apple, or apricots to the cereal if desired.

3. 2 Whole wheat Pancakes (page 151) which may be topped with fresh fruits, lemon, or orange juice with honey, chopped nuts, and the LSA mixture.

4. Muffins—banana and walnut or apple flavored (page 148 and 149). I suggest you have 1–2 pieces fresh fruit with 1–2 muffins.

5. Fresh fruit salad using any seasonal fruits. You may add 3–4 tablespoons of LSA (page 146) as this will give you protein and extra fiber. You may also add 4–5 tablespoons Fruit and Nut Cream (page 146) if desired.

6. Golden Fruit Salad (page 186) sprinkled with 2 tablespoons LSA.

7. Rusher's Shake (page 144) is great if you want a light, quick, and easily digested breakfast.

8. Sweet Rice: 1 bowl cooked brown rice (around 2½ ounces) with wheatgerm and 3 tablespoons LSA. Add soy milk and fresh fruit such as bananas and strawberries, or raisins. You may also add Fruit and Nut Cream (page 146).

9. Savory Rice: 1 bowl cooked brown rice with Mushroom Sauce (page 112). Add side salad of bell pepper, cherry tomatoes, carrot sticks, and celery. You may also add 2–3 dried tomatoes if you like the taste.

10. Scrambled Tofu (page 152) with a side salad of cherry tomatoes, carrot sticks, and sliced apple.

LUNCHES—SECTION THREE

You may have any of the following:

1. Mixed Bean Salad (page 124) sprinkled with LSA, with Garden Fresh Green Salad (page 126).

2. Sandwiches using whole wheat bread, sour dough, rye bread, stone ground bread, rice bread, corn bread, herb and olive bread, walnut bread, or any high-quality bread from the health food store. You may spread the bread with avocado, tahini, or Hummus (page 147). Do not use any butter or margarine.

    For sandwich fillings use finely grated raw carrot, raw zucchini, raw beet and raw winter squash, and you may add canned fish such as sardines, tuna, or red or pink salmon if desired.

    Another healthy and tasty sandwich filling is Tofu Spread (page 147).

    Other suggested sandwich fillings are tofu with grated carrot and golden raisins; tuna with grated carrot, lettuce and red onion rings; strips of free-range chicken, tomato, onion, lettuce, and chopped fresh mint; sliced free-range hard-boiled eggs with lettuce and cucumber; sliced avocado with steamed broccoli and a dash of balsamic vinegar or salt-reduced soy sauce; tahini, grated carrot, and dried apricots.

    To add flavor to sandwiches you may use freshly ground black pepper or lemon pepper, chopped coriander/cilantro, chives or scallions/green onions.

3. Pumpkin Soup (page 140) with 1 slice toast spread with tahini and topped with chopped coriander, chives and parsley.

4. Chicken Soup à la Madeleine (page 141) garnished with a side salad of lettuce, celery, bell pepper, and sliced carrots.

5. Melon and Chicken Breast Salad (page 131).

6. Avocado, Orange, and Mushroom Salad (page 119) with 1 small bowl brown rice sprinkled with LSA.

7. Spinach Salad with Sesame Seeds (page120) with 3 ounce canned tuna or red salmon.

8. Warm Salad of Cherry Tomatoes and Onions (page 121) with 1 bowl Pumpkin Soup (page 140).

9. Green Beans in Ginger Salad (page 121) with 1 bowl brown rice and 1 baked potato.

10. Sprout Salad (page 122) with tuna or red salmon.

11. Spicy Seafood Salad (page 123) followed by 1 orange peeled and quartered.

12. Tabbouleh (page 125) with grilled fish of choice or 1 free-range half chicken breast.

13. Rice Harvest Salad (page 127) with fresh garden salad.

14. Cauliflower and Broccoli Florets with Herb Vinegar (page 127), 2 hard-boiled free-range eggs and 1 slice toast.

15. Potato and Leek Soup (page 134) with 2 slices toast spread with Hummus (page 147) or tahini, sprinkled with LSA.

16. Mumma's Minestrone (page 135) with 2 slices toast or rice cakes spread with tahini or Hummus (page 147) and sprinkled with LSA.

17. Navy Bean Soup (page 136) sprinkled with LSA and served with a fresh garden salad.

18. Celery Soup (page134) with 2 rice cakes topped with red salmon or tuna or 1 free-range skinless half chicken breast or drumstick.

19. Asparagus Soup (page 136) with 1 bowl brown rice sprinkled with LSA or 2 hard-boiled eggs and 2 slices toast.

20. Pita Pizza (page 168) with fresh garden salad and dressing of choice.

21. Terrific Tuna, Tomatoes, and Pasta (page 169) with fresh garden salad and dressing of choice.

22. Spaghetti with Chili Tomato Sauce (page 160) with fresh garden salad and dressing of choice.

23. Whole wheat pasta with a selection of mixed vegetables stir-fried with garlic, onions, reduced-salt soy sauce or tomato paste, freshly ground black pepper, and chili (optional).

24. You may have any one of our yummy salads (see recipes pages 119 to 132) and salad dressings (see recipes pages 114 to 118), with 2 slices toast, or 2 crackers, or rice cakes.

EVENING MEALS—SECTION THREE

You may have any soup (see recipes pages 133 to 143) **or** any dessert (see recipes pages 178 to 186) with any of the following main courses. Do not have more than 2 courses for the evening meal (i.e. don't have a soup and main course and dessert which would be 3 courses as this will overwork the liver and slow down digestion and metabolism. **Always have a raw vegetable salad with your main course as this will improve digestion**. You may have a light salad dressing if desired. If you have a weak digestive system try slowly sipping 1 small glass of water containing 1 teaspoon apple cider vinegar during the meal.

If you don't have much of an appetite for dinner, skip the main course altogether and just have soup and toast or one of our lovely salads (see recipes pages 119 to 132).

For chicken dishes use only free-range skinless chicken.

You may have any of the following:

1. Vegetable Paella (page 153).

2. Herbed, Steamed Fish Fillets (page 154).

3.   Savory Crepes (page 155) with Crustacean Salad (page 128).

4.   Carrot Sunflower Seed Surprise (page 156) with grilled fish of choice or 1 free-range skinless half chicken breast.

5.   Vegetable Casserole (page 156) with 1 bowl brown rice sprinkled with LSA.

6.   Zucchini and Herb Omelette (page 154).

7.   Spicy Chicken Kebabs (page 157).

8.   Stuffed Potatoes with Baked Beans (page 157).

9.   Winter Squash Baked with Sesame Seeds (page 158) with grilled fish or 1 free-range skinless half chicken breast or drumstick.

10. Whole Fish Chinese Style (page 158).

11. Chicken Chow Mein (page 159).

12. Whole wheat pasta with a selection of mixed vegetables stir-fried with garlic, onions, reduced-salt soy sauce or tomato paste, freshly ground black pepper, and chili (optional).

13. Soya Bean Burgers (page 159).

14. Family Fish Cakes (page 161).

15. Hot Vegetable Curry (page 163).

16. Easy Chicken and Leek Casserole (page 162).

17. Beans with Mushrooms (page 163) with 1 small bowl brown rice sprinkled with LSA.

18. Fried Rice with Shrimp (page 164).

19. Golden Casserole (page 165) with 1 small bowl brown rice sprinkled with LSA.

20. Spicy Shrimp with Brussels Sprouts (page 161).

21. Corn Fritters (page 165) with garden salad.

22. Spicy Chicken Sauce and Pasta (page 166).

23. Scallops with Crushed Sesame Seeds (page 164).

24. Red Lentils with Artichokes (page 167) with 1 bowl brown rice sprinkled with LSA.

25. Ratatouille Kebabs (page 167) with grilled fish or 1 bowl brown rice sprinkled with LSA.

26. Grilled Salmon Cutlets (page 166) with salad and/or steamed vegetables of choice.

27. Salmon and Basil Loaf (page 168) with salad or vegetables.

28. Terrific Tuna, Tomatoes, and Pasta (page 169) with salad.

29. Chicken and Almonds (page 169).

30. Vegetable Ratatouille (page 171).

31. Steamed Fish with Ginger and Scallions (page 170).

32. Buckwheat and Vegetables (page 172).

33. Stir-fried Vegetables with Tahini Sauce (page 174).

34. Fried Rice with Egg and Vegetables (page 177).

WHERE TO FIND OUR
Yummy Recipes

Chapter 9

RECIPES FOR THE LIVER-CLEANSING DIET

GENERAL NOTES

The recipes in the LCD are made with all-natural ingredients and are very low in fat. Furthermore, all damaged and unhealthy fats have been eliminated. If you want to speed up your weight loss you may reduce the amount of oil found in some of the recipes and indeed you may make them all totally free of oil simply by replacing oil with Vegetable or Chicken Stock (page 113) or use Campbells All Natural Vegetable Stock. In a small number of recipes we have suggested various sauces and spices such as soy sauce, tamari, oyster sauce, sambal olek (chili paste) , chili powder or sauce, and other things. Always check that these are free of MSG and if you are sensitive or allergic to any of these sauces, spices, or condiments do not include them in the recipes. If you do not like spicy food these sauces and spices can be replaced with Vegetable Stock (page 113) or Campbell's All Natural Vegetable Stock, or replace them with herbs and fresh natural condiments of your own choice.

SOME NOTES ON PASTA

Whole wheat pastas and spaghetti are very healthy, containing fiber, minerals, vitamins, and complex carbohydrates. Of course, the Italians make the best pastas and you can find Italian brands in food stores. Whole wheat pastas can be made from whole wheat, spelt, kamut, and buckwheat and have less calories and more protein than pastas made from refined flour. Spelt and kamut are ancient forms of wheat, whereas buckwheat is a cereal grass with a long history of use in Europe and Japan.

These whole wheat pastas are darker in color and cook *al dente* in 5–7 minutes which is much quicker than pastas made with refined flour.

To cook the pasta, using a large saucepan, bring to a boil 12 cups of water for each 1 lb pasta. When the water is boiling add a small amount of salt, then the pasta. Stir to keep the noodles separate and cook until just before pasta is done, the residual heat in the pasta will continue the softening process as you drain the pasta and toss it with your chosen sauce. Serve pasta as soon as possible while it is hot.

Pasta is popular and very easy to prepare and is tasty with olive oil, garlic, mushrooms, zucchini, potatoes, and dark greens.

SOME NOTES ON MUSHROOMS

Mushrooms have become very popular over the last few years because not only are they tasty, they are also known to be good for the immune system and are definitely one of nature's anti-ageing foods. Chinese herbalists have been using mushrooms medicinally for thousands of years. They are a good source of selenium which is an anti-oxidant mineral with liver protective properties. Suitable types of mushrooms for consumption are field mushrooms and button mushrooms or the more exotic shiitake, maitake, and reishi mushrooms available fresh and dried from gourmet supermarkets, health food stores and Asian food stores. The dried varieties of mushrooms can be reconstituted by soaking in warm water for an hour before cooking. Mushrooms can be eaten raw in salads, included in many cooked vegetable dishes, and are nice sautéed with garlic and olive oil for pastas. If you eat approximately 5–7 oz of various mushrooms per week it will improve your health, unless of course you are allergic to them! We have included mushrooms in several of our recipes for the Liver-Cleansing Diet.

APPLE CIDER

Where apple cider is referred to in the recipes it is recommended that the non-alcoholic variety be used.

HEALTHY DIPS AND PATE

MUSHROOM PATE
Serves 6

3 cups sliced exotic mushrooms or field mushrooms
1 heaped tablespoon finely chopped garlic
2 tablespoons balsamic vinegar
1 cup walnuts
1 cup lentils
¼ cup cold-pressed virgin olive oil
1 teaspoon fresh thyme
1 teaspoon fresh sage
1 teaspoon fresh oregano

Preheat the oven to 350°F. Mix together the mushrooms, garlic, and vinegar in a bowl then spread on a lightly oiled baking sheet. Roast for 15 minutes and set aside. Toast the walnuts in a dry skillet over medium heat for 5 minutes and set aside. Rinse the lentils well under cold running water then place in a saucepan with 2 cups water, cover and bring to a boil. Boil for 5 minutes, then simmer for 20 minutes and drain. Place mushroom mixture, walnuts, lentils, oil, and herbs in a blender or food processor and purée until smooth. Scrape pâté into a bowl, chill, and serve with rice cakes.

SPINACH AND HERB DIP
Makes 2 cups

1 lb spinach
1 cup fresh parsley
1 cup fresh dill sprigs
1 cup plain soy yogurt
2 tablespoons Dijon mustard
1 tablespoon tahini
freshly ground black pepper
pinch sea salt

Add the well-rinsed spinach and parsley to boiling water and cook 1–2 minutes. Drain greens and, when cool, squeeze to remove moisture. Place greens in a blender, add dill and blend until fine. Add yogurt, mustard, and tahini and blend. Add pepper and salt to taste. Chill and serve with crackers.

ROASTED RED BELL PEPPER and SUN-DRIED TOMATO DIP
Makes 3 cups
This dip is slightly hot, delicious, and healthy

10 sun-dried tomato halves (not stored in oil)
2 roasted red bell peppers (instructions follow)
2 garlic cloves, chopped
1 chili (small or large as desired)
6½ oz canned beans (e.g. adzuki, great northern beans, red kidney beans)
6½ soft tofu
1 teaspoon ground cumin
1 teaspoon dried oregano
¼ cup virgin olive oil
freshly ground black pepper
sea salt

Soak the tomatoes in hot water until soft, then squeeze out moisture. Chop tomatoes and place in a blender, add the roasted bell peppers, garlic, and chili and blend until fine. Add the beans and blend until fine. Add tofu, cumin, and oregano and blend until fine. Slowly add oil while blender is still going and season with black pepper and a dash of sea salt. Chill and serve with crackers

To roast bell peppers: bake in a 500°F oven for 15–20 minutes then place in a paper bag, seal tightly and allow to cook in their own heat for 25 minutes. Remove from bag and slip off skins. Remove seeds. Use the peppers immediately or refrigerate for several days in an airtight container until ready to use.

STOCKS AND SAUCES

SALSA CRUDA—sauce for pasta or rice
Serves 4

6 medium tomatoes
2 teaspoons sesame seeds
1–2 garlic cloves, minced
2 tablespoons extra virgin olive oil
¼ cup chopped fresh basil
1 tablespoon balsamic vinegar
freshly ground black pepper
pinch sea salt

You may add vegetables of choice, such as mushrooms, sliced zucchini, bell peppers, onions, finely chopped leafy greens, and finely sliced boiled potatoes. Mix all the ingredients together then sauté 5–10 minutes in a wok or nonstick frying pan.

SIMPLE TOMATO SAUCE—for pasta or rice
Serves 2

Cook 2 tomatoes with a little water and 1 tablespoon reduced-salt soy sauce and ½ teaspoon sambal olek (chili paste). You may add fresh minced garlic if desired.

TOMATO SALSA—for pasta or rice
Makes 2

Chop 2 tomatoes, 1 small onion, 1 garlic clove, 6 fresh basil leaves, 6 sprigs fresh parsley, 1 red bell pepper. Add ½ teaspoon sambal olek (chili paste). Simmer gently and serve with pasta.

MUSHROOM SAUCE—for pasta or rice
Makes 2

Using a nonstick pan, lightly brush the base and sides with cold-pressed virgin olive oil, add 6 button finely sliced mushrooms, a little water, and 1 tablespoon reduced-salt soy sauce. Simmer over a low heat. You may add a little garlic if desired.

TAHINI SAUCE
Serves 4

5 tablespoons tahini
4 tablespoons lemon juice
1 garlic clove, minced
pinch sea salt
pinch chili powder
1 tablespoon sweet chili sauce
7–8 tablespoons purified water
1 tablespoon soy milk yogurt

Combine the tahini, lemon juice, garlic, salt, chili powder, chili sauce and mix thoroughly. As the mixture thickens add the water and beat until sauce runs freely off spoon. Add the yogurt and beat. Mixture should be smooth and easy to pour.

VEGETABLE STOCK

2 carrots	1 turnip
2 onions	1 rutabaga
2 leeks	1 potato
4 large stalks and leaves celery	3 zucchini

Other vegetables can be used. Chop all vegetables, add to a large stock pot with 12 cups water, bring to a boil, simmer for 2 hours and strain. Store the stock in the refrigerator or freeze. Alternatively, Campbell's All Natural Real Vegetable Stock is available from supermarkets and is a good substitute.

CHICKEN STOCK
1 free-range chicken, skinned
4 stalks celery
2 onions, finely chopped
2 leeks, finely chopped
2 carrots, chopped
freshly ground black pepper to taste
2 garlic cloves, chopped
1 heaped tablespoon chopped fresh ginger root

Place all the ingredients in a large saucepan with about 12 cups water, cover and bring to a boil. Reduce heat and simmer slowly for 2 hours. Cool overnight and remove any fat from surface. Strain, then store the stock in the refrigerator or it can be frozen in small containers for future use.

To make **basic fish stock** replace chicken with whole fish of your choice (snapper, perch, whiting). You will need to pass through a sieve to remove fish pieces and bones before refrigerating.

Alternatively, Campbell's All Natural Real Chicken Stock is available from supermarkets, but if possible it is preferable to make your own chicken stock.

SALAD DRESSINGS

ITALIAN DRESSING
2 tablespoons Italian or French wine vinegar
1 garlic clove, minced
pinch sea salt
freshly ground black pepper
5 tablespoons cold-pressed virgin olive oil
2 heaped tablespoons finely chopped fresh parsley

Combine vinegar, garlic, salt and pepper, gradually whisk in the oil and garnish with parsley.

VINAIGRETTE
2 teaspoons mustard (hot English, wholegrain or mild)
2 teaspoons tarragon
2 garlic cloves, minced
½ cup cold-pressed peanut oil
1 tablespoon honey
freshly ground black pepper to taste
½ cup vinegar (apple cider, balsamic or white-wine vinegar)

Place all ingredients, except vinegar, in a bowl and mix well. Then slowly add vinegar to taste, maybe a little more or less according to your preference.

WALNUT DRESSING
2 teaspoons Dijon mustard
pinch sea salt
freshly ground black pepper to taste
2 tablespoons vinegar (apple cider, balsamic, or white-wine vinegar)
½ cup cold-pressed walnut oil
1 tablespoon cold-pressed safflower oil

Combine mustard, salt, pepper, and vinegar in a bowl and gradually whisk in oil.

DILL and LIME DRESSING
4 tablespoons lime juice
2 tablespoons No Oil Italian Dressing (see below)
2 heaped tablespoons freshly chopped dill

Combine all ingredients in a screw-top jar and shake well.

NO OIL ITALIAN DRESSING
1 cup unsweetened apple juice
¼ cup lemon juice
1 teaspoon dried oregano
½ teaspoon dried thyme
½ cup apple cider vinegar
2 garlic cloves, minced
½ teaspoon paprika

Mix ingredients in a blender and refrigerate overnight.

NO OIL FRENCH DRESSING
juice of 1 lemon
¼ cup apple cider vinegar
2 garlic cloves, minced
½ teaspoon dried dill
½ cup purified water
¼ cucumber, very finely chopped
1 teaspoon freshly ground black pepper
2 teaspoons chopped fresh parsley

Mix ingredients in a blender and refrigerate overnight.

AVOCADO and PEPPERCORN DRESSING
1 large avocado, peeled and stoned
1 heaped tablespoon canned green peppercorns, drained and crushed
2 heaped tablespoons orange juice
1 teaspoon grated orange zest
2 tablespoons cold-pressed virgin olive oil

Purée all ingredients in a blender.

LEMON and GARLIC DRESSING
1 cup lemon juice
2 garlic cloves, minced
½ teaspoon mustard

Blend all ingredients in a blender or mix well and serve with a salad.

HERB DRESSING
½ cup No Oil French Dressing (page 115)
1 tablespoon finely chopped garlic chives
2 garlic cloves, minced
1 heaped tablespoon finely chopped fresh dill
1 heaped tablespoon finely chopped fresh mint
1 heaped tablespoon finely chopped fresh coriander/cilantro
1 heaped tablespoon finely chopped fresh basil

Place in a blender and mix. These herbs are good for your liver.

PARSLEY and MINT DRESSING
4 teaspoons lemon zest
¼ cup cold-pressed virgin olive oil
½ teaspoon paprika
2 teaspoons shoyu (Japanese soy sauce)
4 tablespoons purified water
5 tablespoons finely chopped fresh mint
5 tablespoons finely chopped fresh parsley
2 heaped tablespoons finely chopped fresh garlic chives

Place all ingredients in a screw top jar, shake to mix all together, then refrigerate for several hours so flavors can integrate. This dressing is delicious with pasta salads.

EGG-FREE MAYONNAISE

¼ cup ground almonds
1 teaspoon mustard powder
pinch paprika
2 tablespoons lemon juice
2 tablespoons soy milk
pinch sea salt
1 teaspoon freshly ground black pepper
½ cup cold-pressed virgin olive oil

Place all ingredients, except the oil, in a blender and blend until well combined, then add the oil, drop by drop, until half has been used. Add the remaining oil in a fine stream until a creamy mix is formed. This will not be quite as thick as mayonnaise made with eggs.

CREAMY MAYONNAISE

2 large egg yolks
2 teaspoons vinegar (apple cider, balsamic, or rice vinegar)
2 teaspoons lemon juice
½ teaspoon mustard powder
pinch paprika or cayenne pepper
pinch sea salt
¾ cup cold-pressed virgin olive oil

Place all the ingredients, except the oil, in a blender and blend until well combined. Then, with the blender still operating, add half the oil, drop by drop, until mixture is becoming creamy. The rest of the oil can be added more quickly in a fine stream. Should the mixture curdle add 1 teaspoon of either very hot or icy cold water and this should make it revert back to a smooth consistency.

AVOCADO DRESSING
Makes approximately 2 cups

1 ripe avocado, peeled and stoned
1 small garlic clove, minced
¼ cup purified water
2 teaspoons cold-pressed virgin olive oil
2 tablespoons of one of our mayonnaises
1 tablespoon honey

1 tablespoon freshly chopped dill
pinch sea salt
freshly ground black pepper to taste
2 tablespoons fresh lemon juice

Cut the avocado into large cubes and place in a blender with all the other ingredients. Blend until smooth.

BEET DRESSING
1 raw beet, washed, with skin removed and grated
1 cup sunflower seeds
1 cup purified water
juice 2 lemons
2 tablespoons grated lemon zest
2 tablespoons tamari
pinch cayenne pepper
freshly ground black pepper to taste
pinch sea salt
1 garlic clove, minced
2 heaped tablespoons finely chopped fresh basil

Place all ingredients in a blender with the exception of the herbs and process. Prior to serving, add herbs and mix in well.

TOMATO and BASIL DRESSING
6 large ripe tomatoes
½ cup almonds
juice 1 lemon
½ avocado, peeled and chopped
4 scallions/green onions, finely sliced
1 garlic clove, minced
½ cup finely chopped fresh basil leaves
1 teaspoon tamari

Peel the tomatoes and blend with the rest of the ingredients in a blender. Dilute with water to obtain required consistency.

KAYE BELL'S LOVELY SALAD DRESSING
1 tablespoon wholegrain mustard
1 teaspoon honey

5 tablespoons balsamic vinegar
juice ½ orange
1 egg
7 tablespoons cold-pressed virgin olive oil

Place all the ingredients, except the oil, in a blender and mix. Add oil, drop by drop, and mix in to obtain creamy consistency.

SALADS

AVOCADO, ORANGE, and MUSHROOM SALAD
2 tablespoons lemon juice
1 large ripe avocado, peeled and chopped into large chunks
3–4 large oranges, peeled and segmented.
1 iceberg lettuce, finely chopped
6 oz fresh button mushrooms, thinly sliced and marinated (instructions follow)

Marinade:
5 tablespoons freshly squeezed orange juice
2 heaped tablespoons finely grated lemon zest
pinch sea salt
freshly ground black pepper

Place the lemon juice, avocado, and oranges into a bowl, then toss together with lettuce and marinated mushrooms.

To marinate mushrooms mix together the orange juice, lemon zest, and salt and pepper in a bowl, add the mushrooms and leave to stand for at least 1 hour.

WATERCRESS and AVOCADO SALAD
Serves 4

3 ripe avocados peeled and diced (set aside and sprinkle with fresh lemon juice)
1 cup thinly sliced mushrooms
3 cups chopped watercress
1 onion, finely chopped

2 garlic cloves, minced
½ cup chopped chives and parsley, mixed
pinch sea salt
freshly ground black pepper to taste

Place all the ingredients in a bowl, mix together and serve with
Vinaigrette (page 114).

SPINACH SALAD with SESAME SEEDS
Serves 4

1 bunch small leaf spinach
4 tablespoons sesame seeds
2 tablespoons cold-pressed virgin olive oil
1 tablespoon lemon juice
1 teaspoon reduced-salt soy sauce
dash of Tabasco or sambal olek (chili paste)
8 oz cannned water chestnuts, drained and sliced
8 button mushrooms, sliced
2 tablespoons LSA (page 146)

Remove stems and devein the spinach, wash thoroughly and dry in a
clean dishcloth. Place in the refrigerator in the dishcloth to crisp.
Toast the sesame seeds in a pan over moderate heat, shaking constantly. Remove from the pan and let cool. Mix the oil, lemon juice,
soy sauce, and Tabasco as dressing. Place the torn spinach leaves in
a salad bowl and coat with the dressing. Then add the chestnuts and
mushrooms on top of leaves and sprinkle with toasted sesame seeds
and LSA.

TOMATO and BASIL SALAD
1 lb firm ripe tomatoes, thinly sliced
grated zest of 1 lemon
freshly ground black pepper
1 tablespoon lemon juice
2 tablespoons cold-pressed virgin olive oil
pinch sea salt
½ teaspoon honey
6 scallions/green onions, finely sliced
1 cup finely chopped fresh basil

Arrange the tomato slices in a shallow bowl, sprinkle with the lemon zest and pepper. To make the dressing, beat the lemon juice with oil, sea salt, and honey. Place the scallions/green onions and basil over the tomatoes and sprinkle with the dressing. Refrigerate for 1 hour before serving.

WARM SALAD of CHERRY TOMATOES and ONIONS
1 tablespoon cold-pressed virgin olive oil
2 tablespoons honey
1 heaped tablespoon finely chopped fresh oregano
1 heaped tablespoon finely chopped fresh tarragon
1 heaped tablespoon finely chopped fresh basil plus extra for garnish
1 onion, sliced
6 scallions/green onions
2 cups cherry tomatoes (red or yellow)
2 tablespoons Vinaigrette (page 114)

Heat the oil, stir in honey and herbs, add onion slices and increase heat to brown the onions, stirring constantly. Lower heat when onions are colored and add tomatoes, stir gently for approximately 2 minutes, keeping tomatoes whole. Serve warm sprinkled with the Vinaigrette and extra chopped basil.

GREEN BEANS in GINGER SALAD
½-inch piece ginger root, finely grated
1 teaspoon ground fennel
1 lb green beans, trimmed and sliced diagonally
2 heaped tablespoons finely chopped fresh mint
2 heaped tablespoons finely chopped fresh chives
1 teaspoon cold-pressed virgin olive oil

Place 2 cups water into a saucepan, add the ginger and fennel and cook for 2–3 minutes. Add the beans, mint and chives and stir gently. Cook until the beans are just tender. Drain and refrigerate. Toss in oil before serving.

AVOCADO SALAD with PECANS
1 red butter lettuce
3 avocados, peeled and sliced
juice ½ lemon

4 tablespoons Walnut Dressing (page 115)
½ cup pecans

Wash and dry the lettuce and place into a bowl. Add avocados, lemon juice and dressing, fold nuts through salad and toss well.

SPROUT SALAD

4 stalks celery
1 seeded cucumber
10 scallions/green onions, cut diagonally
12 button mushrooms, sliced thinly
1 red Delicious apple, cored and cut into strips
2 tomatoes, peeled, seeded, and chopped
2 cups mixed sprouts (e.g. mung bean, soya bean, and alfalfa)
1 cup mixed salad herbs of your choice (e.g. parsley, chives, basil, dill, coriander/cilantro, etc.)

Combine all the ingredients and toss with one of our salad dressings. Serve on shredded lettuce.

BAMBOO SHOOTS, CARROT, and RAISIN SALAD

1 cup bamboo shoots
1 cup grated raw carrot
1 cup finely sliced radish
1 cup diced scallions/green onions
½ cup raisins
1 heaped tablespoon finely grated orange zest

Combine all the ingredients and toss with one of our salad dressings.

ORIENTAL SALAD
Serves 6

4 oz snow peas, topped and tailed
½ Chinese cabbage, finely shredded
5 tablespoons mung beans
8 oz mung bean sprouts
14 oz canned whole baby corn spears, drained
4 oz fresh button mushrooms, thinly sliced
½ red bell pepper, julienned

10 scallions/green onions, julienned, retaining most of the green parts

Steam snow peas for 2 minutes and plunge into cold water for about 30 seconds. Drain, then combine with all the other ingredients and the special dressing.

Special dressing:
2 tablespoons cold-pressed virgin olive oil
1 tablespoon vinegar (white-wine, balsamic, or apple cider)
juice of 1 lemon
1 tablespoon reduced-salt soy sauce
1 garlic clove, minced
1 heaped tablespoon almond slivers
2 heaped tablespoons toasted sesame seeds

Mix all the ingredients together and pour over the Oriental salad. Toss and serve.

SPICY SEAFOOD SALAD
Serves 2–4

1 lb sea scallops
1 lb cooked peeled shrimp
4 oz snow peas
3 stalks celery, finely chopped
1 red bell pepper, julienned
6 scallions/green onions
14 oz canned sliced water chestnuts

Poach the scallops in boiling water for 2 minutes and remove with a slotted spoon, Set aside to cool. Steam snow peas for 2 minutes then plunge into iced water for 30–40 seconds to stop overcooking. Drain snow peas. Mix all the ingredients in a bowl and toss with special dressing. This salad is nice with cold rice.

Special dressing:
1 garlic clove, minced
4 tablespoons vinegar (apple cider, balsamic, or white-wine)
2 tablespoons cold-pressed virgin olive oil or canola oil
1 tablespoon cold-pressed sesame oil

1 heaped tablespoon dry mustard powder
4 tablespoons reduced-salt soy sauce
pinch chili powder (if desired)

Combine all ingredients for the dressing in a screw top jar and shake vigorously.

MIXED BEAN SALAD
½ cup dried chickpeas
½ cup dried red kidney beans
½ cup dried butter beans
½ cup dried black-eyed beans

Soak all the beans for 12 hours, then wash and drain. Fill a saucepan with cold fresh water, add the beans and bring very slowly to a boil—approximately 30 minutes. Simmer over a low heat for 40 minutes until tender. Rinse, drain, and refrigerate while preparing the special dressing.

Special dressing:
¼ cup cold-pressed virgin olive oil
2 tablespoons lemon juice
1 garlic clove, minced
3 scallions/green onions, finely chopped
1 teaspoon dry mustard
fresh parsley, finely chopped
LSA (page 146)

Mix the first 5 ingredients well, then pour over cold beans and toss. Sprinkle with parsley and LSA before serving. This salad is nice with brown rice or grilled fish.

One of our other dressings may be used if preferred.

BAKED BEET SALAD
4 large beets
4 teaspoons cold-pressed virgin oil
2 large red onions

Preheat the oven to 350°F. Cut the stems from the beets, wash, dry, and wrap each beet in foil, adding ½ teaspoon oil to each packet before sealing. Cut a deep cross into base of each onion but do not peel, and prepare as for beets. Place the beets and onions on a baking tray and bake for 1½ hours or until tender. Allow to cool slightly then peel and cut beets into julienne strips. Peel and slice onion crosswise and then into quarters. Combine in a bowl and cover with the special dressing while still warm. Serve warm or chilled with grilled fish or grilled free-range skinless chicken.

Special dressing:
4 tablespoons raspberry or red-wine vinegar
4 tablespoons cold-pressed virgin olive oil
2 teaspoons caraway seeds
freshly ground black pepper

Mix all ingredients together.

MUSHROOMS with WALNUTS and WALNUT OIL DRESSING
8 oz small button mushrooms
7–10 tablespoons vinegar (apple cider, balsamic or white-wine)
1 tablespoon cold-pressed walnut oil
2 teaspoons Dijon mustard
freshly ground black pepper
pinch sea salt
1 teaspoon date and apple chutney, or chutney of choice
5 tablespoons finely chopped walnuts

Clean the mushrooms, remove stalks, and slice finely. Mix together the vinegar, oil, mustard, pepper and salt, and chutney, then add walnuts and chill. Coat the mushrooms with dressing just prior to serving.

TABBOULEH
¼ cup bulghur
2 tomatoes, peeled, seeded and finely chopped
4 scallions/green onions, peeled and finely chopped
1 cup finely chopped fresh parsley
½ cup finely chopped fresh coriander/cilantro

Combine all ingredients and chill for 1 hour before serving with the special dressing.

Special dressing:
½ cup soy milk yogurt
½ small cucumber, seeded and grated
2 heaped tablespoons finely chopped parsley
2 heaped tablespoons finely chopped chives
2 tablespoons lemon juice
2 tablespoons vinegar (apple cider, or balsamic)

Combine all ingredients and chill.

AVOCADO, MANGO, and LIME SALAD
2 red butter lettuces, washed and torn
1 avocado, peeled and chopped
1 fresh mango, peeled and diced
1 small green bell pepper, finely chopped
1 small red bell pepper, finely chopped
6 scallions/green onions, finely chopped
1 heaped tablespoon finely chopped fresh parsley
1 heaped tablespoon finely chopped fresh chives

Arrange the lettuce leaves on a platter. Combine all other ingredients and mix together with the special dressing. Place on top of lettuce.

Special dressing:
½ cup No Oil French Dressing (page 115)
¼ cup freshly squeezed lime juice
1 garlic clove, minced
1 heaped tablespoon dried tarragon
1 heaped tablespoon finely chopped fresh coriander/cilantro
freshly ground black pepper to taste

Combine all ingredients and mix well.

GARDEN FRESH GREEN SALAD
½ lettuce, washed and torn
10 small spinach leaves, washed and torn
½ romaine lettuce, washed and torn
½ cup snow pea sprouts
1 cup finely chopped watercress
½ cup finely chopped fresh dill

1 red onion, finely chopped
1 garlic clove, minced
4 tablespoons fresh coriander/cilantro
juice of ½ lime
2 heaped tablespoons parsley

Combine all ingredients and serve with one of our lovely dressings.

RICE HARVEST SALAD
½ cup brown rice
½ cup basmati rice
2 corn cobs
½ cup finely chopped dried apricots
½ cup finely chopped dried figs
1 tablespoon LSA (page 146)
¼ cup pine nuts

Boil the brown rice for 20 minutes, add the white rice, boil for a further 10 minutes or until cooked. Drain and cool.

Cook the corn for 15 minutes, then strip corn off cobs. Toast the pine nuts on a nonstick baking tray until golden.

Mix all the ingredients except the pine nuts into the rice, add one of our dressings, and sprinkle with pine nuts.

CORN and RICE DELIGHT SALAD
2 cups cooked brown rice, cold
2 cups cooked corn kernels
1 cup celery pieces
1 cup walnuts
1 cup grated carrot
5 scallions/green onions, finely sliced
2 heaped tablespoons toasted sesame seeds

Combine all ingredients and serve with one of our lovely dressings.

CAULIFLOWER and BROCCOLI FLORETS with HERB VINEGAR
½ cauliflower, broken into florets
3 cups broccoli florets
3 slices lemon
¼ cup each finely chopped mint and parsley
2 cups herb or tarragon vinegar

Lightly cook the cauliflower and broccoli in boiling water with slices of lemon. Drain. Remove the lemon then plunge vegetables into icy water for 30–40 seconds to prevent overcooking. Drain well. Sprinkle with mint and parsley and toss in herb vinegar. Chill for 2–4 hours and toss again. Drain and serve. Alternatively, any of our other dressings may be used if you prefer them to herb vinegar.

CHERRY TOMATO, AVOCADO, and GRAPEFRUIT SALAD

1 radicchio lettuce
1 medium avocado, peeled and diced
1 grapefruit, peeled and divided into small segments
2 cups cherry tomatoes
¼ cup chopped chives

Place the lettuce leaves on a plate and arrange avocado, grapefruit and tomatoes on top. Choose one of our lovely salad dressings and pour it over prior to serving. Garnish with chives.

CRUSTACEAN SALAD

Any cooked seafood, such as crayfish, shrimp, crabmeat, lobster or a mixture of these, may be used in this recipe.

1 heaped teaspoon Madras curry powder
2 tablespoons Mayonnaise (page 116)
soy milk, if desired
1 mango, peeled and mashed
1 heaped tablespoon finely chopped chives
1 heaped tablespoon finely chopped fresh dill
2 lb fresh cooked seafood
1 lettuce, washed and crisped in refrigerator

Stir the curry powder into mayonnaise. If the mixture is too thick add 1 tablespoon soy milk. Add mashed mango, chives, and dill. Stir well. Shell seafood. Make boats from lettuce leaves and top with the seafood and mango mayonnaise.

TUNA and PASTA SALAD

1 lb spiralli pasta
5 tablespoons Vinaigrette (page 114)
6 oz canned tuna in water

2 heaped tablespoons capers
1 green bell pepper, diced
20 fresh basil leaves
2 cups each red and yellow cherry tomatoes
1 red onion, finely chopped

Cook the pasta in 12 cups boiling water until tender—about 10 minutes. Drain and place in a large bowl. Add Vinaigrette, toss in tuna and remaining ingredients and mix well.

POTATO SALAD

6 large potatoes, steamed in jackets
4 hard-boiled free-range eggs
10 scallions/green onions, finely sliced
2 gherkins, finely chopped
½ cup chopped fresh chives
pinch sea salt
freshly ground black pepper
1 cup Mayonnaise (page 117)

Cool potatoes and cut into chunks. Mix gently with all other ingredients.

POTATO and VEGETABLE SALAD

10 small new potatoes with skins on
freshly ground black pepper
pinch sea salt
¼ teaspoon paprika
2 tablespoons cold-pressed virgin olive oil
2 cups broccoli florets with small amount of stem left
6 cups of washed lettuce, dried and torn into small pieces
2 cups coarsely chopped spinach
1 cup alfalfa sprouts
1 cup finely sliced red cabbage

Cook the potatoes for approximately 20 minutes until almost tender. Drain, cool, cut into chunks and place in bowl. Add pepper and salt, paprika, and oil and toss well. Preheat the oven to 400°F. Place the potato mixture on parchment paper suitable for a hot oven. Place on top shelf and bake for 5–10 minutes. Meanwhile, steam the broccoli for 5 minutes or until tender without losing color. Remove from heat and plunge into very cold water for 30–40 seconds to prevent over-cooking, then drain well. Place the lettuce and spinach in a bowl, add sprouts and cabbage. Cut the broccoli lengthwise and add to greens. Add ½–1 cup Mayonnaise (page 116 or 117). Remove the potatoes from the oven and add to the salad.

ASPARAGUS SPEARS and LETTUCE SALAD

1 butter lettuce, washed and crisped in refrigerator
1 red leaf lettuce, washed and crisped in refrigerator
1 red butter lettuce, washed and crisped in refrigerator
3 bunches fresh asparagus
1 red onion, finely sliced

Wash and dry all lettuce leaves then tear into bite-sized pieces removing stalks. Chop thick bases off asparagus and steam on high for 5 minutes. After cooking, plunge asparagus into icy water for 30–40 seconds then drain well. Cut asparagus into bite-sized pieces. Combine all ingredients and toss with one of our dressings (French Dressing is nice).

COLESLAW

1 cup grated carrot
3 cups shredded cabbage (center stalks removed)
1 cup diced green apple
½ cup raw peanuts
½ cup sunflower seeds
½ cup raisins
½ cup finely sliced red bell pepper

Toss all ingredients with one of our lovely dressings. It is nice with Mayonnaise (page 116 or 117).

ZUCCHINI SALAD

8 small zucchini
1 red onion, finely chopped
1 green bell pepper, finely sliced
1 red bell pepper, finely sliced
Cut zucchini into 2-inch slices and steam over boiling water until just tender. Drain and place in a serving dish. Toss with the other ingredients and a dressing of your choice.

PASTA SALAD with AVOCADO

7 oz pasta shells (whole wheat, if possible)
1 tablespoon vinegar (apple cider, balsamic, or white-wine)
2 tablespoons cold-pressed virgin olive oil
freshly ground black pepper to taste
pinch sea salt
1 large ripe avocado
juice and finely grated zest of 1 lemon
2 garlic cloves, minced
2 teaspoons warmed honey
6 scallions/green onions, finely sliced
2 heaped tablespoons each finely chopped parsley and chives

Bring 8 cups water to a boil, add salt and pasta and cook until tender, drain and place in a serving bowl. Blend vinegar, oil and seasoning, pour over pasta and toss. Mash avocado flesh with lemon juice and zest, garlic, and honey. Add scallions/green onions, parsley, and chives then add to pasta and stir lightly.

MELON and CHICKEN BREAST SALAD
Serves 3–4

4 free-range skinless boneless half chicken breasts
1 cup Chicken Stock (page 113)
2 apples, cored and diced
juice of 1 lemon
3 stalks celery
2 dozen green seedless grapes
3 tablespoons Mayonnaise (page 117)
2 cantaloupes, chilled
alfalfa sprouts, for garnish
toasted slivered almonds, for garnsh

Place the chicken breasts and stock in a pan, bring to a boil then simmer on very low heat for approximately 10 minutes. When cooked, remove from pan and cool, then slice into julienne strips. Set aside and chill.

Sprinkle the apples with lemon juice and combine with the celery and grapes, fold in the chicken strips. Add the mayonnaise.

Place the peeled, seeded and sliced cantaloupes in the center of a plate and arrange the chicken mixture on top. Decorate with alfalfa sprouts and toasted slivered almonds.

APPLE, CARROT, and BEET SALAD

1 large Granny Smith apple
2 carrots
1 medium beet
juice of ½ lime
2 tablespoons cold-pressed olive oil
pinch sea salt
freshly ground black pepper
½ teaspoon honey
1 red butter lettuce
1 butter lettuce

Grate the apple, carrots, and beet. Place the lime juice, oil, salt, pepper, and honey into a screw-top jar and shake. Arrange washed and dried lettuce leaves on plates. Place some of the grated mixture into the center of each leaf. Spoon dressing over the top.

SNOW PEA SALAD

2 cups snow peas
1 red butter lettuce
1 large ripe avocado, peeled and diced
2 cups cherry tomatoes, halved
¼ cup alfalfa sprouts
4 sprigs fresh basil, finely chopped

Top and tail the snow peas and steam for approximately 3 minutes until just tender, then plunge into icy water for 30–40 seconds to prevent overcooking. Drain. Tear the washed and dried lettuce leaves into bite-sized pieces and arrange in the bottom of a salad bowl. Add avocado, tomatoes, snow peas, sprouts, and basil. Choose one of our lovely salad dressings and pour over the salad.

SOUPS

NOODLE SOUP
Serves 4

15 oz spinach, washed and chopped
15 oz celery, chopped
16–20 fresh asparagus spears, cut into 1-inch pieces
4 cups Vegetable Stock (page 113) or Campbell's All Natural Stock
1 tablespoon cold-pressed virgn olive oil
½ teaspoon cumin
½ teaspoon dried basil
½ teaspoon sea salt
15 oz noodles

Place the vegetables in a medium-sized saucepan with the stock. Bring to a boil and add all remaining ingredients, except for the noodles. Lower heat and cook for 10 minutes. Cool and purée half of this mixture in a blender and then return to the saucepan. Add the noodles and cook for an additional 7 minutes.

HARICOT BEAN SOUP
Serves 4

6½ oz haricot (Navy) beans
small slice lemon
8 cups Chicken or
    Vegetable Stock (page 113)
1 onion, chopped
2 carrots, chopped
2 leeks, chopped
2 stalks celery, chopped
7 oz tomatoes
⅔ cup chopped parsley
freshly ground black pepper

Soak the beans in water for 4 hours. Drain. Using fresh water, cook the beans with the lemon slice until tender—approximately 45–60 minutes—then drain, reserving liquid. Brush the base of a saucepan with oil and add ¼ cup of the stock. Add the onion and cook gently for 2 minutes. Add the carrots, leeks, and celery and cook for 5 minutes. If desired skin the tomatoes (easier when placed in boiling water for a few minutes), then chop and add them to the other vegetables. Cook for a further 5 minutes adding more stock if required. Heat the remaining stock and make up to 8 cups with the reserved liquid from the beans. Bring to a boil then simmer for 30 minutes or until the vegetables are soft, then add the beans and reheat. Stir in the parsley and black pepper just prior to serving.

POTATO and LEEK SOUP
Serves 4

1 lb potatoes, peeled and sliced
4 leeks, well washed and sliced into 1-inch pieces
1 teaspoon finely chopped fresh dill
1 teaspoon finely chopped fresh mint
8 oz scallions/green onions, chopped
2 tablespoons finely chopped parsley

Boil the potatoes and leeks for approximately 15 minutes in 4 cups water. When cool, transfer potatoes, leeks and cooking water plus dill and mint to a blender and purée until smooth. Place back on a low heat, add scallions/green onions and cook for a further 10 minutes. Serve sprinkled with the parsley.

CELERY SOUP
Serves 4

5 cups Vegetable Stock (page 113) or Campbell's All Natural Stock
3 leeks, chopped
1 lb celery with leaves, chopped
2 potatoes, peeled and chopped into cubes
1 tablespoon lemon juice and finely grated zest of 1 lemon
1 cup water
additional cup finely sliced celery

Combine all the ingredients, with the exception of the finely sliced celery, in a large saucepan and simmer for 2 hours. Cool, then purée and return to soup pan. Add the cup of finely sliced celery and stir through. Simmer for 5 more minutes and serve.

VEGETABLE and BARLEY SOUP
Serves 4–6

1 cup barley   1 cup chopped green beans
6 cups water   13 oz canned tomatoes

2 cups chopped carrot
1 cup chopped onion
2 garlic cloves, minced
½ small rutabaga, grated
2 cups grated parsnip

2 tablespoons tomato paste
2 tablespoons vinegar
 (apple cider, or white-wine)
1 teaspoon dried marjoram

In a large saucepan, cook the barley in the water until soft, but not overcooked, about 15–20 minutes. Remove approximately half the barley with a slotted spoon and place in a blender. Blend with a little of the liquid until smooth. Return this to the pan. Add the carrot, onion, garlic, rutabaga, parsnip, and beans. Cook until the vegetables are tender, then stir in the tomatoes, tomato paste, vinegar, and marjoram. Cook slowly for approximately 60 minutes.

MUMMA'S MINESTRONE
Serves 4–6

2 large onions, chopped
2 garlic cloves, minced
10 cups Vegetable or Chicken
 Stock (page 113)
2 large carrots
4 stalks celery and leaves
2 large leeks (use whole leek)
2 large potatoes
3 small zucchini
10 green beans

1 cup sliced mushrooms
28 oz canned tomatoes
(Optional)1 teaspoon finely
 chopped sambal olek (chili paste)
freshly ground black pepper
3 cups cooked haricot or Navy
 beans (instructions follow)
1 cup cooked brown rice or
 whole wheat macaroni
2 teaspoons dried marjoram

In a large saucepan cook the onions and garlic for 6 minutes in ½ cup of the stock. Add the remaining stock, vegetables, tomatoes and sambal olek. Season with black pepper. Bring to a boil and simmer for 1–2 hours stirring occasionally.

When cool, purée 3 cups of the soup in a blender and return to pan. Add the haricot or Navy beans, rice or macaroni, and marjoram and heat for a further 5 minutes.

To prepare haricot beans: soak 1½ cups dried beans in water for 4 hours. Drain. Using fresh water with a slice of lemon, cook the beans for approximately 45–60 minutes until tender.

CHILLED SUMMER BEET SOUP
Serves 4–6

4 cups puréed cooked beets
4 cups Vegetable Stock (page 113) or Campbell's All Natural Stock
5 tablespoons finely chopped garlic chives
2 teaspoons finely grated lemon zest
freshly ground black pepper to taste

Combine all ingredients and mix well. Chill. To serve, garnish with scallions/green onions, garlic chives and grated raw beets.

NAVY BEAN SOUP
Serves 6–8

2 cups beans (navy, great northern or, pinto)
10 cups water
2 tablespoons cold-pressed virgin olive oil
¼ cup tamari
2 onions, diced
6 garlic cloves, diced
pinch sea salt
freshly ground black pepper
1 teaspoon finely chopped red bell pepper
1 carrot, sliced
1 stalk celery, sliced
2 bay leaves

Cover the beans with water and soak overnight. Rinse and place in a large pot, cover with fresh water and place over a medium heat. Add the oil, tamari, one of the diced onions, 3 of the garlic cloves and salt and pepper and cook for 1 hour. Add the bell pepper, carrot, celery, remaining onion and garlic cloves, and bay leaves. Cook for approximately 1 hour, until the carrots and beans are tender.

ASPARAGUS SOUP
Serves 4–6

16½ fresh asparagus spears **OR**
    12 oz canned asparagus and liquid

3 cups Chicken or Vegetable Stock (page 113)
1 cup finely chopped celery leaves
3 large potatoes, peeled and chopped
1 tablespoon lemon juice

If using fresh asparagus cook in boiling water for 4 minutes. Drain, retaining the cooking liquid. Combine all ingredients, except for 6 of the asparagus spears, with ½ cup of the retained asparagus liquid and cook for 1 hour. When cool, purée in a blender until smooth. Reheat gently and serve, using the retained asparagus spears to decorate the soup.

TOMATO SOUP
Serves 6–8

1 tablespoon cold-pressed virgin olive oil
4 garlic cloves, minced
4 onions, diced
2 celery stalks, sliced
10 cups tomato stock (tomato juice or cooked tomatoes squeezed
    through a strainer)
½ cup tamari
1 teaspoon each dried basil, dried oregano, garlic powder
pinch sea salt
4 tablespoons soy powder
2 tablespoons cornstarch
½ cup finely chopped fresh parsley

Heat the oil in a wok, add the garlic and onion and sauté for 5 minutes. Add the celery and sauté for 3 minutes. Add the stock and seasonings. Cook for 30 minutes over low heat. Dilute the soy powder in 2 cups of stock and add to the soup. Add the cornstarch and re-season to taste. Cook for a further 30 minutes over a low heat. For a better infusion of flavors make this soup the day before you wish to serve it. Add parsley just prior to serving.

LEEK AND LENTIL SOUP à la Florentine
Serves 4

½ cup red lentils

2 teaspoons salt-reduced soy sauce
1 heaped tablespoon dried basil
1 teaspoon dried oregano
1 tablespoon cold-pressed virgin olive oil
1 large leek (white part only), chopped and well washed
2 carrots, chopped
2 cups chopped broccoli
6 cups pure water

On low heat, gently fry the lentils, soy sauce, basil and oregano in the oil, stirring constantly. Add the chopped vegetables. Stir until vegetables are slightly fried then add the water and simmer for 1 hour, adding more water if required. For variation, place ½–¾ soup in blender and purée, returning puréed soup to the saucepan. Garnish with parsley to serve.

SPLIT PEA SOUP
Serves 6

8 cups green split peas
8 cups Vegetable Stock (page 113) or Campbell's All Natural Stock
1 onion, diced
2 garlic cloves, minced
2 bay leaves
2 celery stalks, diced
2 large carrots, diced
1 turnip, diced
1 potato, diced
⅓ cup tamari
1 teaspoon each garlic powder, dried basil, dried marjoram
pinch sea salt
¼ cup barley

Combine the peas and stock in a large saucepan and bring to a boil over a medium heat. Reduce heat and add the onion, garlic, bay leaves, celery, carrot, turnip, potato, tamari, and seasonings. Cook for 1 hour until peas and vegetables are soft. Remove the bay leaves. When cool, transfer the soup to a blender and blend until smooth. Pour back into the pan, add the barley and cook a further 2 hours, stirring often.

SOUP of FRUIT
Serves 2

8 oz strawberries
2 apples
juice of 1½ oranges
1 tablespoon finely grated lemon zest

Purée the strawberries in a blender then place into a saucepan. Grate the apples and add to strawberries with the orange juice and lemon zest. Bring to a boil, then simmer for 10 minutes. Remove from the heat and put through a sieve. Discard residue and return the mixture to the saucepan to reheat. If desired, the mixture can be thickened with a little cornstarch dissolved in orange juice. Simmer for 3 more minutes, stirring continuously, allow to cool and chill. Serve with slices of orange or strawberries and soy milk yogurt and honey.

BORSCHT
Serves 4–6

4½ cups Chicken Stock (page 113)
4 raw beets, peeled and chopped
2 green apples, cored, peeled, and chopped
5 tablespoons honey
juice of 4 large lemons
1 teaspoon ground allspice
freshly ground black pepper
pinch sea salt
2 egg yolks
chives, for garnish

Place all the ingredients except the egg yolks and chives into a saucepan and cook until the beets are tender. Cool and blend in blender until smooth. In a separate bowl, beat the egg yolks and thicken by adding a little of the hot soup. Then pour the egg yolk and soup mixture back into the main pot of soup, beating to keep it smooth and simmer for15 minutes. Chill the soup and serve cold with chopped chives.

MUSHROOM CONSOMME
Serves 6

2 lb mushrooms, sliced
2 lb onions, chopped
freshly ground black pepper
pinch sea salt
1 teaspoon lemon juice
scallions/green onions, julienned
extra button mushrooms, very finely sliced
watercress sprigs, for garnish

In a large pan place the mushrooms, onions, salt, lemon juice, and 8 cups water. Bring slowly to a boil, reduce heat, cover and simmer gently for approximately 2 hours. Strain through a colander and return to the pan. Add a little salt and pepper to taste and reheat gently. Pour into soup bowls and garnish with the scallions/green onions, finely sliced mushrooms and a few sprigs of watercress.

PUMPKIN SOUP
Serves 8–10

2 small butternut squash, diced
3 cups diced winter squash
2 onions, diced
2 garlic cloves, minced
2 stalks celery, chopped
2 carrots, chopped
6 cups Vegetable Stock (page 113) or Campbell's All Natural Stock
¼ bunch fresh basil
½ cup fresh coriander/cilantro
2 tablespoons soy sauce
pinch sea salt
freshly ground black pepper
3 bay leaves
¼ bunch flat-leaf parsley, chopped
1 cup unflavored non-dairy soy milk

Place the vegetables into a large pot with the stock and herbs. Add soy sauce, salt, pepper, bay leaves, and parsley. Bring to a boil, reduce heat and simmer on a very low heat for 1 hour. Allow to cool, remove bay leaves and blend soup in a blender or food processor until smooth. Add the soy milk in the blender last, and use more if mixture is too thick.

LENTIL SOUP
Serves 2

½ cup lentils, rinsed and drained
4 cups mushroom kombu stock (instructons follow)
1 teaspoon sea salt
2 onions, cut into half moons
2 stalks celery, finely sliced
tamari to taste

Cook the lentils in the stock for ½ hour or until tender, add salt and vegetables and cook until tender. Add tamari during last 10 minutes of cooking. You may serve like this or pass through a blender if preferred.

Mushroom Kombu Stock: Soak 6 shiitake mushrooms in water for 5 minutes. Put a piece of kombu seaweed in 8 cups cold water and put on a high heat. Add the mushrooms and the water they have been soaking in and bring to a boil, reduce heat and simmer for 10 minutes. Remove kombu and place it on a towel to dry. Remove the mushrooms and reserve them for another dish, or if desired you may use them in this lentil soup as they are very good for the immune system. This stock keeps for up to 1 week in the refrigerator.

CHICKEN SOUP à la Madeleine
Serves 4–6

To make the stock:

1 free-range chicken (with skin removed)	celery tops
2 bay leaves	½ cup parsley sprigs
1 large onion	2 garlic cloves

Simmer slowly for 90 minutes under cover, the whole chicken with the bay leaves, onion, celery tops, parsley, and garlic cloves in approximately 3 pints water. Strain the liquid into a soup pot. Keep the chicken and the stock in the refrigerator overnight.

To make the soup:

2 large onions, diced

½ bunch fresh basil

¼ bunch fresh coriander/cilantro

1 cup flat-leaf parsley, chopped

2 cups V8 vegetable juice (optional)

¼ cup pearl barley

½ cup orange lentils

2 bay leaves

2 carrots, finely chopped

6 stalks celery, finely chopped

¼ small Chinese cabbage

1 small parsnip, finely chopped

1 small turnip, finely chopped

1 small sweet potato, finely
    chopped

pinch sea salt

freshly ground black pepper

Place the onions, basil, coriander/cilantro, and parsley in a blender or food processor and blend until smooth. Take the chicken from refrigerator and remove bones and fat. Cut the chicken meat into bite-sized pieces. Skim fat from the top of the stock pot and add the V8 vegetable juice to the stock pot. Add the pearl barley and lentils to the stock with bay leaves and simmer until tender. Chop all vegetables finely and add to the pot. Cover and simmer for approximately 1 hour, then add the chicken pieces. Season with sea salt and black pepper.

MINESTRONE SOUP à la Madeleine
Serves 4

2 brown onions, peeled

½ bunch of fresh basil

¼ bunch fresh coriander/cilantro

½ bunch of flat-leaf parsley

1 large can V8 vegetable juice or 6 cups Vegetable Stock (page 113)

2 tablespoons soy sauce

2 vegetable stock cubes (free of MSG)

13 oz canned tomatoes

½ cup brown lentils

½ cup pearl barley

4 bay leaves

2 garlic cloves

2 stalks celery with leaves, finely chopped

2 carrots, finely chopped

½ parsnip, finely chopped

1 small turnip, finely chopped
freshly ground black pepper to taste
1 can red kidney beans (wash thoroughly)

Place the onions, basil, coriander/cilantro, and parsley in a food processor or blender and blend until finely chopped.

In a large soup pot place the vegetable stock or V8 juice, soy sauce, 1 cup hot water, and stock cubes mixed with 1 cup warm water. Stir and add the onion and herb mix from the blender. Place the tomatoes in the food processor and blend, add to soup pot. Add the lentils, pearl barley, and bay leaves. Cover and cook on low heat. Pass the garlic through a garlic press and add to pot. Chop finely the celery, carrots, parsnip, and turnip, add to the pot. Cover and cook slowly for 80 minutes stirring occasionally, season with black pepper if desired. Add the kidney beans and cook for another 10 minutes.

BREAKFASTS

DRINKS AND SHAKES

SUMMER PUNCH
1 cup carrot juice
½ cup apricot nectar
¼ cup pineapple juice
crushed ice and ground nutmeg

Blend juices together, pour over ice and sprinkle with nutmeg.

RUSHER'S SHAKE
Makes 4 cups

1½ cups vanilla or plain soy milk
½ cup crushed ice
1 banana
12 strawberries
1 cup chopped fresh pineapple
1 tablespoon honey
3 tablespoons LSA (page 146)

Blend together and serve immediately.

MELON MAGIC HEALTH SHAKE
½ cantaloupe, cut into chunks
½ honeydew melon, cut into chunks
1 cup chopped watermelon
crushed ice
1½ cups vanilla or plain soy milk
3 tablespoons LSA (page 146)
1 tablespoon honey

Blend together and serve immediately.

NANASTRAWKI SHAKE

1½ cups vanilla or plain soy milk
1 ripe banana
12 strawberries
2 kiwifruit, peeled and diced
2 tablespoons LSA (page 146)
1 tablespoon honey
1 cup crushed ice

Blend together and serve immediately.
Raspberries, blackberries, or blueberries can be added or substituted in this mix.

We have given you these recipes but you are really only limited by your imagination. You may use any fruit combinations you desire. If you have a juice extractor, vegetable juices may be added.

HOMEMADE HEALTHY SPREADS AND ADDITIONS

LSA

LSA stands for Linseeds, Sunflower seeds, and Almonds. To make it, use:

3 cups linseeds (flaxseeds)
2 cups sunflower seeds
1 cup almonds

Mix and grind together until fine. A regular coffee grinder will do the job. Store in an dark airtight glass jar in the refrigerator.

This mixture has a slightly sweet and nutty taste and can be sprinkled on rice, pasta, fruit, vegetables, or just about anything. It is a good source of protein, essential fatty acids, minerals, and fiber and is definitely an anti-ageing mixture.

APRICOT JELLY (makes a good substitute for jams and preserves)

5 oz dried apricots
2 oz golden raisins
3½ oz dried apples
4 cups unsweetened fresh orange juice.

Simmer all the ingredients until fruit is soft. Cool and purée in blender then place in sterilized jars (sterilize with boiling water). Seal when mixture cools and keep in refrigerator.

PINEAPPLE GINGER SPREAD

2 cups unsweetened crushed pineapple, well drained
1 teaspoon minced fresh ginger root

Combine all the ingredients and use to spread on toast.

FRUIT and NUT CREAM

¾ cup fresh raw cashews
¾ cup almonds (blanched or with skins soaked off)
3 oranges, peeled and sectioned
1 apple, peeled and sectioned
1 tablespoon natural honey, if sweet taste desired
Combine. If desired, add some vanilla extract and/or ground nutmeg.

Grind nuts and add to the fruit. Place this mixture in a blender and blend until fine and creamy.

This is nice on top of fresh fruit salad or with pancakes.

TOFU SPREAD

7 oz canned salmon, water-packed
3½ oz tofu
2 scallions/green onions, finely chopped
1 heaped tablespoon finely chopped fresh coriander/cilantro
2 sprigs fresh mint, finely chopped
juice of ½ lemon
freshly ground black pepper

Combine all ingredients, mash to a paste and spread on toast or use as a sandwich filler with cucumber and tomato.

HUMMUS

4 oz dried chickpeas
4 large garlic cloves, chopped
4 tablespoons sesame seeds
juice of 3 lemons
1 teaspoon paprika

Soak the chickpeas overnight and discard skins. Drain. Using fresh water, boil the soaked chickpeas for 1 hour and drain. Place the chickpeas in a blender and blend with the garlic until smooth. Set aside. Place the sesame seeds in a grinder and grind until smooth. Add to chickpeas and garlic. Stir in the lemon juice and mix well. Sprinkle with paprika. Spread on sandwiches, biscuits, or toast instead of butter or margarine.
Note: If preferred, hummus can be bought ready-made at health food stores or supermarkets.

AVOCADO SPREAD

Mash 1 ripe avocado with freshly ground black pepper, 2 finely chopped scallions/green onions and lemon juice to taste.

MUFFINS

APPLE MUFFINS (makes 12 muffins)
1½ cups whole wheat self-rising flour
½ teaspoon mixed spice
½ teaspoon ground cinnamon
½ cup golden raisins
2 egg whites
2 tablespoons cold-compressed almond oil
1 cup chopped cooked apple
1 tablespoon honey or concentrated apple juice
½ cup soy milk

Preheat the oven to 350°. Sift the flour and spices and add golden raisins. Beat the egg whites and add the oil, apple, honey, and soy milk and blend thoroughly. Add to the dry ingredients and stir until thoroughly mixed. Spoon into a lightly greased muffin tin and bake in the oven for 17 minutes, or until cooked.

BANANA and WALNUT MUFFINS à la Madeleine (makes 12 muffins)
5 ripe bananas, mashed
¼ cup cold-pressed canola oil
⅔ cup honey
1 teaspoon vanilla extract
2⅓ cup all-purpose wholewheat flour
¾ teaspoon baking powder
⅔ cup chopped walnuts
½ teaspoon salt
¾ teaspoon ground nutmeg
1 teaspoon baking soda

Preheat the oven to 350°F. Lightly oil a 12-cup muffin pan. Stir together the bananas, oil, honey, and vanilla in a bowl. In another bowl combine the flour, baking powder, walnuts, salt, nutmeg, and baking soda. Stir the wet ingredients into the dry mixture and blend with a spoon. Spoon this mixture into muffin cups, filling to the rim. Bake until golden brown—about 20–25 minutes. Serve warm.

BANANA and WALNUT MUFFINS à la Wendy

Makes approximately 8 muffins

2 ripe bananas, mashed
2 tablespoons honey
2 tablespoons cold-pressed virgin olive oil
1 heaped tablespoon LSA (page 146)
2 teaspoons vanilla essence
1¼ cups whole wheat self-rising flour
2 tablespoons walnuts

Preheat oven to 350°F. Mix the bananas, honey, oil, and LSA in a large bowl. Fold in remaining ingredients and mix. Spoon into a nonstick muffin pan and bake in the oven for approximately 20–25 minutes.

CRANBERRY and MANDARIN MUFFINS

2½ cups wholewheat flour
2 teaspoons baking powder
⅔ cup freshly squeezed orange juice
⅔ cup brown rice syrup
⅓ cup honey
¼ cup cold-pressed canola oil
⅔ cup canned mandarin oranges, drained
¾ cup thawed frozen or fresh cranberries

Preheat the oven to 350°F. Lightly oil a 12-cup muffin pan. Combine the flour and baking powder in a bowl. In another bowl mix together the orange juice, rice syrup, honey, oil, and mandarin oranges. Add the dry mixture to the wet mixture and mix. Stir in the cranberries. Spoon this mixture into muffin cups, filling to the rim and bake until golden brown—about 20–25 minutes. Serve warm.

SOYA BEAN BURGERS

Makes approximately 12 burgers

13 oz canned or cooked soya beans, drained and coarsely blended
  with 1 tablespoon tahini
2 stalks celery, chopped
1 carrot, grated
1 onion, finely chopped

2 garlic cloves, minced
2 heaped tablespoons chopped fresh parsley
1 heaped tablespoon garlic chives, chopped
1 heaped tablespoon coriander/cilantro
1 egg
½ cup cooked buckwheat or wild rice
freshly ground black pepper
pinch sea salt
1 tablespoon sesame seeds

Mix all the ingredients together except the sesame seeds. Add some whole wheat all-purpose flour if the mixture is too runny. Using an ice-cream scoop, form patties and roll each one in sesame seeds. Refrigerate for 30 minutes. Cook in a nonstick pan, which has been brushed on the base and sides with cold-pressed oil, until golden brown, then flip over.

Serve plain or with Mushroom or Tomato Sauce (page 112).

CEREALS

You may have 1½–1¾ oz Special K, Raisin Bran, oatmeal, or unsweetened and untoasted meusli. Do not use cows' milk, instead use soy, almond, or rice milks.

There is also another lovely milk called Amasake which is a sweet fermented rice beverage. Amasake is Japanese—it may be available from specialty food stores.

If you prefer you can make your own muesli using:

2 cups rolled oats	½ cup seedless raisins
1 cup rye flakes	½ cup sunflower seeds
½ cup chopped dried dates	¼ teaspoon ground nutmeg
½ cup shelled walnuts	¼ teaspoon ground cinnamon
½ cup almonds	4 cups apple cider

Combine and mix all ingredients except the cider in a large bowl. Place in an airtight container and stir in cider, seal and refrigerate overnight. Serve with soy milk, rice milk, or almond milk.

Fresh fruit, such as bananas, strawberries, prunes, kiwifruit, oranges, apples, or any fruit of your choice may be added to any low-fat wholegrain cereal.

JAFFLES OR TOASTED SANDWICHES

Heat jaffle iron and brush lightly with cold-pressed virgin olive oil. Place bread slices in jaffle iron and fill with one of suggested fillings. Close and cook for 4–6 minutes.

Some suggested sandwich fillings are baked beans, Mushroom Sauce (page 112) or Cooked Mushrooms (page 152), free-range egg, Hummus (page 147), Tofu Spread (page 147), Pineapple and Ginger Spread (page 146), Apricot Jelly (page 146), salmon, sardines, tuna, tomatoes, onions, garlic, or various combinations of these.

WHOLE WHEAT PANCAKES
Makes approximately 6–8 pancakes

1 whole egg
1 cup soy milk
¾ cup whole wheat self-rising flour
1 teaspoon vanilla extract, if sweet pancakes desired

Beat the egg with half the milk and mix in half the flour, then the rest of the flour and milk alternately. Beat well to remove all the lumps. Let the mixture stand in the refrigerator for 15 minutes. Heat a non-stick pan which has been lightly brushed on the base and sides with cold-pressed virgin olive oil. Use a medium heat and pour ½ cupfuls of mixture into pan. Flip over when bubbles appear on uncooked side.

Fill the pancakes with fresh fruit or citrus juice and honey and sprinkle with LSA (page 146) or chopped raw nuts. You may also have a savory pancake using Mushroom Sauce (page 112), Tofu Spread (page 147), Curried Egg (below) or Grilled Tomato (page 152).

EGGS—healthy ways to cook them for the LCD. Use free-range eggs.

Curried Eggs: Boil 4 eggs for 10 minutes, mash with 2 tablespoons soy milk and 1 tablespoon curry powder and mix well.

Perfect Poached Eggs: Fill a nonstick pan with water, add 1 tablespoon apple cider vinegar and bring to a boil. Add eggs and reduce heat to cook to desired consistency. Make sure there is enough water to cover the eggs.

Hard Boiled or Soft Boiled Eggs are also healthy. Remember never fry eggs as their cholesterol turns to dangerous oxidized 'oxy-cholesterol'.

SCRAMBLED TOFU
Serves 3

2 tablespoons water
1½ lb tofu chopped
2 small onions, peeled and diced
1 tablespoon minced garlic
½ green bell pepper, finely chopped
½ cup fresh mushrooms, sliced
4 tablespoons cold-pressed virgin olive oil
1 tablespoon brown mustard
2 tablespoons white miso or soy sauce
2 teaspoons curry powder
2 tablespoons finely chopped fresh mint or parsley
1 teaspoon dried tarragon
½ teaspoon chili powder
¼ teaspoon freshly ground black pepper
½ teaspoon sea salt

Heat the water in a skillet or wok, add the tofu, onions, garlic, bell pepper and mushrooms, then add oil. Cook for 8–10 minutes over a medium heat. Mix the mustard and miso together in a bowl and pour over the tofu mixture in the wok. Stir in the curry powder, mint, tarragon, chili powder, black pepper, and salt and continue cooking for 6–8 minutes until most of the liquid in the wok evaporates. Serve hot with a salad, vegetables, or toast. You may sprinkle with LSA (page 145) to increase the protein content.

GRILLED TOMATOES
Halve the required number of tomatoes, then make small slits in each tomato half and place a sliver of garlic in each. Lightly brush with cold-pressed virgin olive oil and grill.

COOKED MUSHROOMS
As many finely sliced button or field mushrooms as desired.

Heat a nonstick pan which has been lightly brushed on the base and sides with cold-pressed virgin olive oil, add water and mushrooms, then reduced-salt soy sauce and soy or rice milk. Cook on a low heat.

MAIN COURSES

WILD RICE STUFFED TOMATOES
Serves 4

8 medium tomatoes
1 cup cooked wild rice
1 onion, finely chopped
⅔ cup currants
4 tablespoons chopped pine nuts
2 heaped tablespoons chopped mint
2 heaped tablespoons chopped chives
freshly ground black pepper to taste
½ cup whole wheat bread crumbs
1 heaped tablespoon LSA (page 146)

Preheat the oven to 350°F. Remove the tops from the tomatoes and scoop out the pulp with a metal spoon. Combine the rice, onion, currants, pine nuts, mint, chives and tomato pulp in a saucepan and season with black pepper. Bring the mixture to a gentle simmer and cook for 1 minute. Place the tomato cases on a foil-lined baking tray. Spoon the mixture into tomatoes and sprinkle breadcrumbs and LSA over each tomato. Bake in the oven for 20 minutes.

VEGETABLE PAELLA
Serves 4

1½ cups brown rice
2 cups Chicken or
    Vegetable Stock (page 113)
2 large onions, sliced
2 leeks, julienned
3 carrots, sliced
2 zucchini, sliced thickly
2 garlic cloves, minced
1 red bell pepper, sliced

2 tablespoons tomato paste
1 teaspoon turmeric
4 tomatoes, peeled and chopped
freshly ground black pepper to
    taste
8 oz broccoli, broken into florets
8 oz cauliflower, broken into
    florets

Parboil the rice in the chicken stock for 20 minutes. Set aside but do not drain. Add onions, leeks, carrots, zucchini, and garlic to a non-stick pan and cook for 10 minutes in 5 tablespoons water over medium heat. Add bell pepper, tomato paste, turmeric, and tomatoes and cook for 2 minutes. Add rice with stock and stir until combined with all ingredients and simmer gently for approximately 15 minutes. Separately cook broccoli and cauliflower for 5 minutes and add to the above just before serving.

HERBED, STEAMED FISH FILLETS
Serves 4

4 fillets or cutlets of snapper, mackerel, blue-eyed cod or bass

Seasoning:
2 cups breadcrumbs
2 heaped tablespoons finely chopped coriander/cilantro
2 heaped tablespoons finely chopped parsley
2 heaped tablespoons finely chopped chives
1 heaped tablespoon finely chopped basil
2 tablespoons chutney
1 tablespoon seeded mustard
1 egg white

Push a sharp-bladed knife through the center of each fillet lengthwise to make a pocket for stuffing. Combine the seasoning ingredients and place into the pocket of each fillet. Secure the ends with tooth picks. Add a small amount of water to a nonstick frying pan and cook fish over high heat for 5 minutes on each side.

ZUCCHINI and HERB OMELETTE
Serves 1

2 free-range eggs
1 zucchini, grated
2 scallions/green onions, finely sliced
2 heaped tablespoons finely chopped parsley
2 heaped tablespoons finely chopped chives
freshly ground black pepper to taste

Combine all the ingredients, mix well and pour into a nonstick omelette pan. Cook until mixture is firm, then turn omelette over and cook the other side. Serve with one of our salads.

DOLMADES—STUFFED VINE LEAVES
Makes approximately 40

8 oz preserved vine leaves rinsed in hot water
juice of ½ lemon
2 tablespoons cold-pressed virgin olive oil

Filling:
1 cup long-grain rice
1 tablespoon cold-pressed virgin olive oil
1 large onion, finely chopped
2 heaped tablespoons pine nuts
2 heaped tablespoons chopped parsley
2 heaped tablespoons currants, washed
freshly ground black pepper

Lay the vine leaves flat on a cutting board shiny side down. Set aside any torn leaves. To make filling, wash the rice well and drain. Heat the oil and fry onion until soft. Add the pine nuts and fry until golden. Take off heat and add the rice and remaining ingredients. As the vine leaves are salty no added salt is necessary. Put a spoonful of filling onto each vine leaf and roll up. Line the base of a saucepan with damaged leaves. Place the stuffed leaf parcels on top, close together and seam side down. Cover with an inverted plate. Pour over the lemon juice, olive oil, and enough water to just cover the plate. Cover the pan, bring to a boil, reduce heat and simmer for 40 minutes. Remove and check that rice is tender. Cool in the liquid. Can be served warm or chilled.

SAVORY CREPES
Serves 4

1 cup stoneground whole wheat all-purpose flour
1 teaspoon dry mustard
1¼ cups soy milk
3 egg whites

Combine all the ingredients in a blender and blend until smooth. Let stand for 30 minutes. Pour a little mixture onto the hot surface of a nonstick pan or crepe maker, rotate pan quickly to distribute the mixture evenly and pour off any excess. As bubbles appear, turn crepe to brown on the other side. These very fine crepes take only a very short time to cook so take care not to burn them.

CARROT SUNFLOWER SEED SURPRISE
Serves 4

1 large onion, finely chopped
2½ cups sliced carrots
¾ cup water
freshly ground black pepper to taste
1 tablespoon honey
¼ cup soy grits (ground soya beans)
2 heaped tablespoons finely chopped dill
¼ cup sunflower seeds
2 free-range egg whites, lightly beaten
¼ cup chopped almonds

Preheat the oven to 350°F. Place onion and water in a saucepan and bring to a boil, add carrots and cover. Simmer until carrots are tender. Stir in all the other ingredients with the exception of the almonds. Pour into a shallow baking dish, sprinkle with almonds and bake in the oven for 20 minutes.

VEGETABLE CASSEROLE
Serves 6–8

4 large potatoes, peeled and cut into chunks
2 carrots, cut into large chunks
1 parsnip, peeled and cut into chunks
½ rutabaga, cut finely
1 cup chopped celery
1 cup green peas
1 cup green beans
26 oz canned tomatoes, drained
2 cups unsweetened orange juice plus 1 tablespoon orange zest
3 cups Vegetable Stock (page 113) or Campbell's All Natural Stock
4 tablespoons LSA (page 146)
freshly ground black pepper to taste

Preheat the oven to 350°F. Place all ingredients in an earthenware casserole dish, cover and cook in the oven for 2 hours. This dish is ready when the vegetables are tender and the liquid has reduced to a sauce. If desired, you may thicken with a small amount of cornstarch.

SPICY CHICKEN KEBABS
Serves 4
Marinade:
1 garlic clove, minced
2 teaspoons finely grated fresh ginger root
2 heaped tablespoons finely chopped fresh coriander/cilantro
½ cup lemon juice

2 free-range skinless boneless half chicken breasts, cut into cubes
2 large onions, cut into pieces suitable to place securely on skewer
1 large mango, sliced
12 mushrooms, whole or halved depending on size
1 green bell pepper, seeded and cut into pieces suitable for skewer

Mango Sauce:
1 fresh mango, peeled and chopped
1 heaped tablespoon parsley, finely chopped
1 garlic clove, minced
1 teaspoon fresh grated ginger
pinch chili powder
1 teaspoon allspice
1 tablespoon honey

Combine all marinade ingredients and marinate chicken overnight.

Arrange chicken pieces with other ingredients alternately on skewers. Grill or barbecue until chicken becomes golden.

Blend all sauce ingredients in a blender until fine. Serve with the kebabs. Sauce can be served hot or cold.

STUFFED POTATOES with BAKED BEANS
Serves 4–6

1 large scrubbed potato per person
2 heaped tablespoons chopped scallions/green onions
2 heaped tablespoons chopped chives
2 heaped tablespoons chopped parsley

3 tablespoons LSA (page 146)
13 oz canned baked beans

Preheat the oven to 400°F. Bake the potatoes with their skins on in a
hot oven for 1½ hours. Remove and cut in half lengthwise. Scoop out
potato flesh and place into a bowl with the scallions/green onions,
chives, parsley, and LSA and mash well. Add the baked beans and
mix in. Refill potato cases with this mixture and return to the oven
until heated through. Vary the amount of ingredients according to the
number of potatoes required.

WINTER SQUASH BAKED with SESAME SEEDS
Preheat the oven to 400°F. Cut the winter squash into serving pieces
and steam until just tender. Brush each piece with a little cold-
pressed virgin olive oil and sprinkle with sesame seeds. Place in the
oven and cook until tender.

WHOLE FISH CHINESE STYLE
1 whole fish (snapper or trout) weighing approximately 2¼ lb
¼ cup lemon juice
5–6 cups Chicken or Fish Stock (page 113)
1 medium onion, diced
1 stalk celery, diced
1 carrot, julienned
1-inch piece ginger root, finely chopped
2 garlic cloves, minced
garnish (instructions follow)

Clean and scale the fish then rub inside and out with lemon juice.
Place the stock in a wok or large deep frying pan and add vegetables,
ginger, and garlic. Arrange a rack with chopsticks or place an
upturned bowl in the base of the wok. Bring the stock to a boil over
a low heat and place the fish on the rack. Pour over 1 cup of the stock
and flavorings. Steam for 20–30 minutes, or until cooked. Or wrap
fish in foil and bake at 350°F in oven for 25 minutes while simmering
the stock for 20–30 minutes.

Place the fish on a heated serving dish and bring the remaining
stock to a rapid boil until slightly reduced and spoon over the fish.
This dish can be served hot or cold.

To make garnish: peel a carrot and cut into matchstick strips. Slice finely 2 scallions/green onions. Soak the carrots and scallions/green onions for 1 hour in ½ cup balsamic vinegar and ½ cup unsweetened orange juice. Drain and sprinkle over the fish to garnish.

CHICKEN CHOW MEIN
Serves 6

6 cups Chicken Stock (page 113)
4 tablespoons brown rice
2 onions, chopped
1 cup chopped celery
1 cup sliced carrots
1 cup green beans
1 small bok choy
1 cup cauliflower
1 cup broccoli
2 teaspoons curry powder
1 teaspoon Chinese five spice powder (free of MSG)
2 teaspoons grated ginger root
1 lb steamed chicken pieces
2 cups noodles

Bring the stock to a boil, reduce heat and add all ingredients except the chicken and noodles. Simmer for approximately 20 minutes. Cook the noodles by boiling for 3 minutes, drain and rinse well. Add the chicken and noodles to the stock mixture and heat through. Can be thickened if desired with cornstarch.

SOYA BEAN BURGERS
Serves 4–6

1 lb dried soya beans
4 tablespoons LSA (page 146)
2 medium onions, chopped
1 heaped tablespoon chopped parsley
1 cup mashed potato
1 cup egg white
2 tablespoons tomato sauce
2 tablespoons salt-reduced soy sauce
½ teaspoon ground nutmeg

freshly ground black pepper
whole wheat all-purpose flour
whites of 3 eggs beaten with 2 tablespoons soy milk
1 cup whole wheat breadcrumbs

Place the beans in a saucepan and cover with water to 1 inch above level of beans. Bring to a boil and cook for 1 minute. Remove from heat, do not drain, cover and allow to stand for 1 hour. This is the equivalent of overnight soaking. Cook the beans in the same liquid for 2½ hours or until beans are tender. Drain and mash beans well and add LSA. Combine with the onions, parsley, potato, cup of egg white, tomato and soy sauce, nutmeg, and pepper. Use an ice-cream scoop to form into patties. Coat each patty with flour, dip into egg white and milk mixture and coat with the breadcrumbs. Brush sides and base of a nonstick pan with olive oil and fry patties on both sides until golden brown.

SPAGHETTI with CHILI TOMATO SAUCE
Serves 6

1 large onion, chopped
1 green bell pepper, sliced
2 stalks celery, chopped
½ cup mushrooms
2 garlic cloves, minced
1 cup sliced carrots
14 oz canned tomatoes and juice
½ cup tomato paste
1 cup water or Vegetable Stock (page 113)
2 heaped tablespoons finely chopped fresh basil
2 teaspoons dried or fresh oregano
2 bay leaves
freshly ground black pepper
1 teaspoon chili paste or dash chili powder (optional)
seafood of choice (optional)
1 packet whole wheat spaghetti

Stir-fry the onion, bell pepper, celery, mushrooms, garlic, and carrots in ¼ cup water for 6 minutes. Add all other ingredients, except spaghetti, and cook gently for ½ hour. You may add cooked seafood if desired such as shrimp, scallops, oysters, lobster, octopus, etc.

Cook the spaghetti, combine with sauce and serve with garden-fresh salad and crusty bread.

FAMILY FISH CAKES
Makes approximately 12 cakes

4 large potatoes, peeled
freshly ground black pepper to taste
6 scallions/green onions, finely chopped
8–10 oz fish (canned tuna or salmon, or cooked fillets of any fish
    can be used)
2 carrots, grated
1 stalk celery, finely chopped
1 unbeaten egg white
1 extra egg white and 1 tablespoon water, beaten together
whole wheat fresh breadcrumbs and LSA

Boil the potatoes until tender, drain, add pepper and scallions/green onions and mash well. Add the fish, carrots, celery, and unbeaten egg white and mix thoroughly. Leave mixture to cool then with an ice-cream scoop, make mixture into patties. Dip each patty into egg white and water mixture and roll in breadcrumbs and LSA. Place the fish cakes in the refrigerator for 2 hours. Dry-bake the cakes in a frypan for 5 minutes on each side, or lightly brush cakes with cold-pressed virgin olive oil and grill on foil.

SPICY SHRIMP with BRUSSELS SPROUTS
1 lb brussels sprouts, trimmed with an X cut into each stem end
2 tablespoons cold-pressed peanut oil or virgin olive oil
10 whole scallions/green onions, chopped, (keeping white and green
    ends separately)
2 garlic cloves, minced
2 heaped tablespoons finely grated ginger
2 lb green shrimp, shelled and deveined
1 teaspoon minced red chili peppers (optional)
1 teaspoon sambal olek (chili paste)
1 teaspoon mild chili powder (optional)
1 teaspoon sesame oil
4 tablespoons water
Cook the brussels sprouts, uncovered, in boiling water for 8 minutes

then place under very cold water for 30–40 seconds to prevent over-cooking. Drain. Cut crosswise into ¼-inch slices.

Heat the oil in a wok over medium heat and add the whites of the scallions/green onions. Cook these for 1 minute then stir in the garlic and ginger and cook for a further 3 minutes. Add the shrimp and hot peppers (if desired) and cook, tossing constantly until the shrimp turn pink, about 3–4 minutes.

Combine the sambal olek (chili paste), chili powder (if desired), sesame oil, and water in a small bowl. Stir this into the shrimp mixture and cook 1 minute. Add the brussel sprouts and cook until warmed through. Add the green tops of the scallions/green onions and re-heat. Serve with brown rice.

Note: If you do not like hot spicy food leave out chili powder and hot peppers.

EASY CHICKEN and LEEK CASSEROLE (STEW)
Serves 4

6 free-range skinless, boneless half chicken breasts
1 teaspoon chili sauce
6 leeks, julienned
2 cups celery, cut into chunks
3 medium potatoes, peeled and cut into chunks
2 cups finely sliced carrot
6 cups Chicken Stock (page 113)
13 oz canned tomato pieces in juice
freshly ground black pepper to taste
½ cup chopped parsley

Steam the chicken breasts, cut into chunks and place in a flameproof casserole dish. Add the chili sauce, leeks, celery, potato, and carrot to the chicken and pour over the chicken stock. Bring to a boil then simmer for 20 minutes or until the vegetables are tender. Add the tomatoes, pepper, and parsley. Cover and simmer for another 30 minutes. The casserole may be thickened with a small amount of cornstarch mixed with some of the cooled stock.

HOT VEGETABLE CURRY

Serves 4

2 cups Vegetable Stock (page 113)
1 teaspoon turmeric
1 teaspoon chili powder
1 teaspoon ground ginger or freshly grated ginger
1 teaspoon coriander/cilantro
1 cup carrot strips
1 cup zucchini, cut into chunks
1 cup celery, cut diagonally
1 cup green beans, cut into 3 cm lengths
1 garlic clove, minced
1 cup thinly sliced onions
1 cup cauliflower florets
1 cup mixed red and green bell pepper, cut into strips
1 cup sliced mushrooms
2 leeks, well-washed and cut diagonally
12 oz canned whole tomatoes and juice
1 cup finely cut scallions/green onions

Bring the stock and spices to the boil in a large saucepan, then reduce heat. Add the vegetables and simmer until they are just tender but still crisp. Add tomatoes and scallions/green onions and simmer for 10 minutes.

Serve with brown rice, whole wheat pasta, or noodles, sprinkled with LSA.

BEANS with MUSHROOMS
Serves 1

8 oz button mushrooms, finely sliced
8 oz scallions/green onions, finely chopped
8 oz cooked adzuki (Chinese) beans
1 tablespoon cold-pressed virgin olive oil
1 teaspoon tarragon
1 teaspoon dill
freshly ground black pepper to taste

Preheat the oven to 375°F. Lightly grease a small baking dish with sesame or olive oil. Combine all the ingredients and place in the baking dish. Cover the dish with foil or a glass lid and bake in the oven for 25 minutes.

FRIED RICE with SHRIMP
Serves 2–3

1 tablespoon cold-pressed virgin olive oil
4 cups cooked brown rice
6 garlic cloves, diced
1 teaspoon ground ginger or freshly grated ginger
¼ cup tamari
8 cooked shrimp, peeled and finely sliced
8 scallions/green onions, finely chopped

Brush the base and sides of wok or skillet with the oil and add enough rice to cover the bottom. Fry rice for 6 minutes until golden brown, reducing heat to medium and stirring constantly with a spatula. Add small amounts of water as rice gets dry.

Add 1 teaspoon of the diced garlic, half the ginger and season to taste. As each batch of rice is cooked, place in a baking dish. Repeat the process until all the rice is fried. Toss in the shrimp and scallions/green onions and warm through, then serve.

SCALLOPS with CRUSHED SESAME SEEDS
Serves 6

1 lb fresh sea scallops
3 tablespoons crushed or ground sesame seeds
1 small onion, grated
1 garlic clove, minced
freshly ground black pepper
pinch sea salt
1 red bell pepper, finely sliced
12 red cherry tomatoes
12 yellow cherry tomatoes
¼ cup unsweetened pineapple juice

Combine all ingredients and leave to marinate 4 hours. Then thread scallops and tomatoes on skewers and barbeque or grill for 6–10 minutes.

GOLDEN CASSEROLE

Serves 3–4

1 small winter squash (about 1 lb), peeled and cut into chunks
1 lb carrots, peeled and sliced
2 tablespoons cold-pressed virgin olive oil
3 garlic cloves, diced
3 onions, diced
⅓ cup tamari
1 teaspoon dried oregano
1 teaspoon dried basil
1 teaspoon paprika
2 stalks celery, diced
½ cup bran, wheat germ, or bread crumbs
5 tablespoons LSA (page 146) plus extra for sprinkling
½ cup blended raw peanuts

In a large pot combine the winter squash and carrots with 3 cups water and simmer over a medium heat for 20 minutes until tender. Drain, conserving liquid for soup stock. Mash the winter squash and carrots together until smooth. Heat the oil in pan and add diced garlic, onions, seasoning, and celery and cook for 7 minutes until tender. Preheat oven to 350°F. Add the sautéed vegetables to the squash and carrot and mix well. Mix in the bran, LSA, and blended peanuts. If a thicker consistency is required, add ¼ cup all-purpose flour. Transfer mixture into a large baking dish (8 x 12 in), brush the top lightly with oil and sprinkle with LSA. Bake for 35–40 minutes.

CORN FRITTERS
Serves 4

4 large corn cobs
2 eggs (separate yolks and whites)
2 tablespoons all-purpose flour
pinch sea salt
freshly ground black pepper
cold-pressed virgin olive oil

Cut the kernels from 2 of the corn cobs and place them in a medium-sized bowl. Then, using a heavy knife, scrape the cobs over the bowl to extract their juices. Grate the corn from the remaining cobs (i.e.

cut off the kernels at about half their depth and then with the back of the knife's blade, scrape off what is left on the cob), mixing the cut pulp and milk with the kernels.

Beat the egg yolks in a large bowl until light, beat in the flour, salt and pepper and stir in all the corn. Beat the egg whites in a large bowl until stiff and fold them into the corn mixture. Heat a heavy skillet or griddle iron over medium heat and brush it with oil. Drop ¼ cup of the batter at a time onto the hot griddle or pan and cook for about 30–45 seconds per side. Transfer the cooked fritters to a serving platter and keep warm in a low oven while cooking the remainder.

SPICY CHICKEN SAUCE and PASTA
Serves 6

2 lb free-range skinless boneless chicken breasts, ground
1 large onion, diced
1 garlic clove, minced
2 stalks celery, chopped
1 bell pepper, finely chopped
14 oz canned tomatoes
5 tablespoons tomato paste
1 tablespoon dried oregano
1 tablespoon dried basil
1 tablespoon sambal olek (chili paste)
2 tablespoons cold-pressed virgin olive oil
3 cups purified water

Brush the base and sides of a saucepan with oil and heat. Add the ground chicken and brown, then add all the other ingredients and simmer for 3 hours. When mixture reduces add more water.

Serve with whole wheat pasta.

GRILLED SALMON CUTLETS
Lightly brush salmon cutlets with cold-pressed virgin olive oil and sprinkle with fresh dill and lemon juice. Place under a hot grill for approximately 4 minutes on each side. Serve with vegetables or a salad of your choice.

RED LENTILS with ARTICHOKES

Serves 4

1⅓ cups red lentils
4 tablespoons cold-pressed virgin olive oil
2 medium red onions, sliced
2 garlic cloves, minced
28 oz canned artichoke hearts, drained and halved
1 tablespoon finely chopped capers
14 oz fresh tomatoes, chopped
2 heaped tablespoons finely chopped parsley
2 heaped tablespoons finely chopped chives
½ cup water
¼ cup tomato paste
1 tablespoon red-wine vinegar
1 tablespoon honey

Add the lentils to a large pan of boiling water and boil uncovered for 8 minutes or until just tender, then rinse and drain well. Heat half the oil in a wok, add onions and garlic and stir-fry over low heat until soft. Add remaining oil, artichokes, capers, tomatoes, parsley and chives and stir until heated, add lentils and all remaining ingredients and stir until hot. This is nice with a bowl of brown rice sprinkled with LSA or grilled fish of your choice.

RATATOUILLE KEBABS
Serves 3–4

4 tablespoons cold-pressed virgin olive oil
1 garlic clove, minced
1 tablespoon tomato paste
6 zucchini, cut into chunks
12 baby onions, cut in halves
24 button mushrooms, cleaned and stalked
2 red bell peppers, roasted and skinned (page 111)
2 green bell peppers, roasted and skinned (page 111)
12 red cherry tomatoes
12 yellow cherry tomatoes

Mix the olive oil, garlic, and tomato paste until smooth. Brush this mixture onto the vegetables after they have been threaded onto skewers, then barbeque or grill.

PITA PIZZA
Serves 1–2

1 large pita bread
2 tablespoons tomato paste
vegetables (see below)
seafood of choice (optional)

Preheat the oven to 400°F. Finely chop onions, mushrooms, bell pepper, tomatoes, precooked potato scallops (slices of potatoes steamed),
sliced zucchini, and 6 olives. Spread tomato paste over pita bread and
add all the above ingredients, spread a little additional tomato paste
over topping and bake in the oven for 10 minutes. If you are a seafood
lover you may also add precooked seafood, such as sliced shrimp,
scallops, crab meat, or octopus, but make sure it is very fresh. Serve
with fresh garden salad.

SALMON and BASIL LOAF
Serves 4–6

28 oz canned red salmon (drained and flaked)
½ cup fresh whole wheat breadcrumbs
5 tablespoons LSA (page 146)
5 tablespoons tomato paste
2 stalks celery, finely chopped
1 onion, finely chopped
1 heaped tablespoon finely chopped fresh basil
1 heaped tablespoon finely chopped fresh chives
3 free-range eggs, beaten
1 garlic clove, minced (optional, but remember, garlic is a liver
cleanser)

Mix all the ingredients thoroughly. Brush the base and sides of a loaf
tin with cold-pressed virgin olive oil, and fill with the above cold mixture. Refrigerate for 1 hour, then turn the loaf out into an ovenproof
dish and baste with a little more oil. Bake in oven at 350°F for 40
minutes. Serve hot or cold with vegetables or salad of choice.

TERRIFIC TUNA, TOMATOES, and PASTA

Serves 4

1 tablespoon cold-pressed virgin olive oil
8 garlic cloves, minced
1 onion, chopped
28 oz canned tomatoes and juice
2 tablespoons tomato paste
salt and pepper to taste
2 tablespoons chopped fresh basil
2 medium-sized tuna steaks
pinch ground hot chili (optional)
1 lb penne pasta

Heat oil in a nonstick pan and sauté 4 of the garlic cloves and onions
for a few minutes. Add the tomatoes, tomato paste, salt, pepper, and
basil and stir together. Cover and simmer for 20 minutes, but keep stirring to prevent sticking and add a little water if too dry. Set this aside.

In a large heavy-based pan or wok that will hold all the ingredients,
cook the remainder of the garlic in a little oil for 2 minutes. Add the
tuna and cook for 3 minutes each side, then flake the tuna into pieces
with a fork. Add the sauce and ground chili (if desired) and cook for
approximately 5 minutes on medium heat.

Cook the penne until *al dente* and pour the sauce over the pasta.
Serve with a salad and crusty bread.

GRILLED OCEAN PERCH (ORANGE ROUGHY) with FENNEL

Brush the base and sides of a baking tray with cold-pressed oil. Place
branches of fresh fennel sprinkled with 1 chopped onion on the tray.
Lightly brush fish fillets with oil and place on top. Grill and serve with
freshly squeezed lemon juice and vegetables and a salad of your choice.

CHICKEN and ALMONDS
Serves 2–3

1 cup chopped green beans
½ cup diced celery
½ cup chopped red bell pepper
2 tablespoons cold-pressed virgin olive oil
½ cup blanched or skinned almonds
½ cup diced onion

1 lb free-range skinless boneless chicken pieces
1 garlic clove, minced
1 heaped tablespoon finely diced fresh ginger root
½ cup sliced fresh mushrooms
2–3 cups Chicken Stock (page 113)
2 tablespoons cornstarch
3 tablespoons reduced-salt soy sauce
1 spring onion, chopped
10 sprigs fresh coriander/cilantro
¼ cup chopped basil leaves

Steam the beans, celery and bell pepper, starting with the beans, then adding celery and lastly the bell peppers for a few minutes. Set aside. Heat the oil and fry the almonds until golden brown, remove from oil and drain on paper towels. Sauté the onion in the same pan for 2 minutes, then add chicken pieces and sauté for 2 minutes. Add garlic, ginger, mushrooms, stir and sauté for 2 minutes, adding water if the mixture gets too dry. Add 1 small cup chicken stock and cook for 10 minutes. Blend cornstarch with the remainder of the chicken stock and stir slowly into saucepan. Bring to a boil and cook for 3 minutes while stirring. Add the steamed vegetables, soy sauce, spring onion, and fresh herbs.

STEAMED FISH with GINGER and SCALLIONS
Serves 4

1 lb fish fillets (bass, snapper, orange roughy)
8 scallions/green onions
2–inch piece fresh ginger, peeled
½ cup fresh coriander/cilantro sprigs
2 tablespoons reduced-salt soy sauce
2 tablespoons cold-pressed virgin olive oil
juice of ½ fresh lime
juice of ½ fresh lemon

Wash, skin and cut the fish into 2–inch pieces. Arrange fish on a small serving dish and put into a steamer. A large bamboo steamer or a cake rack in the bottom of a wok with a fitted lid also works well. Shred the green scallions/green onions and ginger into thin matchsticks and scatter half of them over the fish, saving the rest for garnishing. Cover well and cook gently over a moderate heat for 5 minutes or until fish flesh turns white. Place the fish on a serving plate, add the remaining ginger, scallions/green onions, and coriander/cilantro and sprinkle with soy sauce. Heat the oil and lemon and lime juice until hot and pour over fish.

STUFFED BELL PEPPERS
Serves 4

4 large green bell peppers
Stuffing:
4 scallions/green onions, finely chopped
4 oz canned tuna in brine, drained
5 tablespoons cooked rice
2 tablespoons LSA (page 146)
freshly ground black pepper
pinch sea salt
Sauce:
4 tomatoes, chopped
4 garlic cloves, minced
1 tablespoon all-purpose flour
¼ teaspoon chili powder (optional)
2 teaspoons dried coriander/cilantro
1 teaspoon ground cumin

Pre-heat oven to 350°F. Wash the bell peppers, slice a lid off each and put lids aside. Scoop out the seeds. Mix the stuffing thoroughly and push into the bell peppers. Put lids back on. Brush the base and sides of a baking tray lightly with cold-pressed virgin olive oil and add 1 tablespoon water. Stand the bell peppers in the tray and bake in a moderate oven until soft, approximately 45 minutes. Blend the sauce ingredients in blender, heat and serve with the stuffed bell peppers.

VEGETABLE RATATOUILLE
Serves 4

large can V8 vegetable juice or 3 cups Vegetable Stock (page 113)
3 tablespoons soy sauce
2 onions, sliced
2 carrots, julienned
4 potatoes, sliced thinly
4 zucchini, sliced thinly

1 small red bell pepper, sliced thinly
1 small green bell pepper, sliced thinly
14 oz canned peeled tomatoes
1 eggplant, sliced thinly
8 black olives
¼ bunch fresh basil, finely chopped
½ cup finely chopped fresh parsley
1 teaspoon dried mixed herbs
freshly ground black pepper
pinch sea salt
8 bay leaves

Preheat the oven to 325°F. Place some V8 juice or vegetable stock in the bottom of a casserole dish with the soy sauce. Place layers of vegetables in the dish and between layers place herbs and pepper and salt. Add stock or V8 juice as you place the layers of vegetables. Place bay leaves down both sides of the dish and cover. Bake in the oven for 1–1½ hours. Serve with brown rice or whole wheat pasta sprinkled with LSA, and a fresh garden salad.

BUCKWHEAT and VEGETABLES
Serves 3–4

2 tablespoons cold-pressed virgin olive oil
1 medium onion, finely chopped
1½ cups roasted buckwheat (from health food store)
1 teaspoon ground cumin
1 teaspoon turmeric
1 medium carrot, diced
1 stalk celery, diced
1 small green bell pepper, finely chopped
1 cup shredded cabbage
freshly ground black pepper
pinch sea salt
2½ cups water
2 garlic cloves, minced
2 tablespoons salt-reduced soy sauce (optional)

Heat the oil in a large frying pan and sauté the onion, buckwheat and spices and, while stirring, add all the finely chopped vegetables. Season with salt and pepper. Stir in the garlic, bring to a boil and reduce heat to low. Add soy sauce for extra taste. Cover and cook for 20–25 minutes.

BAKMI GORENG
Serves 4

(The pieces from the whole chicken left over from making the chicken stock may be used in this recipe)
2 tablespoons chopped scallions/green onions
1 large tomato, chopped
1 garlic clove, minced
1 heaped tablespoon fresh peeled and chopped ginger root
pinch sea salt
freshly ground black pepper
10 fresh coriander/cilantro sprigs
¼ cup chopped fresh basil leaves
4 free-range skinless boneless half chicken breasts, precooked and cut into pieces
3–4 tablespoons cold-pressed virgin olive oil
1 carrot, julienned
1 stalk celery, chopped
¼ cup shredded Chinese cabbage
½ green bell pepper, cut into strips
1 cup Chicken Stock (page 113)
1 lb cooked thin egg noodles

Combine scallions/green onions, tomato, garlic, ginger, salt and pepper, coriander/cilantro, and basil with the chicken pieces and oil (or stock) and sauté for 2–3 minutes. Then add carrot, celery, cabbage, and bell pepper and sauté for a few minutes. Add chicken stock to the mixture with the precooked egg noodles. Reduce heat and simmer 5 minutes, adding more chicken stock if mixture is too thick.

KAYE BELL'S CHICKEN PARADISO
2 onions, finely chopped
1 teaspoon cold-pressed virgin olive oil
1 cup Chicken Stock (page 113)
1 lb free-range skinless boneless chicken breasts, cut into pieces

26 oz canned peeled tomatoes
1 heaped tablespoon chopped fresh basil
2 garlic cloves, minced
1 bay leaf
1 teaspoon dried oregano
freshly ground black pepper
pinch sea salt
1 tablespoon tomato paste

Sauté the onions in the olive oil and chicken stock, then add the chicken pieces. Cook for 10 minutes. Add the tomatoes, basil, garlic, bay leaf, oregano, and seasonings and then the tomato paste. Simmer for 30 minutes. Serve hot with a garden-fresh salad or one of our liver-cleansing salads.

STIR-FRIED VEGETABLES with TAHINI SAUCE

1 onion, finely chopped
1–2 tablespoons cold-pressed virgin olive oil
2 tablespoons salt-reduced soy sauce
1 garlic clove, minced
1 heaped tablespoon freshly chopped ginger root
juice of ½ lime
1 carrot, julienned
20 snow peas, topped and tailed
½ bunch broccoli, broken into small florets
4 scallions/green onions, julienned
7 oz canned baby corns
½ cup fresh mung bean sprouts
2 stalks celery, finely sliced
¼ Chinese cabbage, finely shredded
½ red bell pepper, finely chopped
1 zucchini, finely sliced
2 tablespoons chili sauce (optional)
2 tablespoons MSG-free fish sauce (optional)
1 bunch spinach, finely chopped
½ bunch of fresh coriander/cilantro

Sauté the onion in the oil, then add the soy sauce, garlic, ginger, and lime juice. Add the vegetables, except the spinach, beginning with the carrot. Then add the chili sauce and fish sauce. Stir-fry over a low heat. Add the spinach and chopped coriander/cilantro last and continue cooking for 5 minutes. Serve with the lovely Tahini Sauce (page 113).

NO OIL STIR-FRIED VEGETABLES
Serves 4

1 cup Vegetable Stock (page 113) or Campbell's All Natural Stock
8 cups mixed diced vegetables, such as cauliflower, cabbage, corn kernels, mushrooms, green and red bell peppers, snow peas, broccoli, zucchini, onions, potatoes, carrots
1 teaspoon chili powder (optional)
2 teaspoons MSG-free oyster sauce or soy sauce
2 garlic cloves, minced

Place 3 tablespoons of the stock in a large wok and heat. Stir-fry the vegetables in this until color in vegetables intensifies. Add the remaining stock, chili, oyster or soy sauce, and garlic and stir-fry to heat through. This is nice served with a bowl of brown rice sprinkled with LSA (page 146).

WILD MUSHROOM and CHESTNUT RAGOUT
Serves 12

2 cups dried chestnuts
2 oz dried cèpes or field mushrooms
1 large leek, washed and chopped thinly
3–4 tablespoons cold-pressed virgin olive oil
6 cups white mushrooms, stemmed and thinly sliced
6 cups fresh cremini or other wild mushrooms, stemmed and cut into cubes
6 cups fresh portobello mushrooms, stemmed and cut into cubes
1 cup Vegetable Stock (page 113) or Campbell's All Natural Stock
6 garlic cloves, roasted (instructions follow)
1 teaspoon dried rosemary
pinch sea salt
freshly ground black pepper
chopped fresh flat-leaf parsley, for garnish

Place the chestnuts in a bowl and cover with water to soak overnight. Drain chestnuts and place in a medium-sized saucepan. Add 4 cups cold water, bring to a boil, reduce heat and simmer for approximately 1 hour, until chestnuts are soft. Drain and coarsely chop chestnuts and set aside. Place cèpes or other dried mushrooms in a bowl and cover with warm water. Soak for 30 minutes until soft. Squeeze these mushrooms to remove their moisture and then chop; there should be about 1½ cups. Reserve their soaking liquid. Sauté the leek in oil for 5 minutes, stir in the white mushrooms and cook for 8 minutes. Add the chopped cèpes or other dried mushrooms and cook over low heat for 10 minutes. Add cremini and portobello mushrooms and cook for 10 minutes, stirring constantly to avoid burning. Cook until the mushrooms are tender. Add the vegetable stock to the pot and simmer for 5 minutes. Stir in roasted garlic, rosemary, and 1 cup of the reserved cèpes soaking liquid. Add the cooked chestnuts and keep stirring, adding more cèpes liquid if needed to keep the mixture moist. Season with salt and pepper to taste. Serve hot and sprinkle with parsley sprigs. This ragout can be cooled and refrigerated in an airtight container for 2 days. Reheat the ragout in a covered pot until hot.

This mushroom dish is nice with brown rice or pasta. If you have trouble getting all the fancy mushrooms, just do your own version of this dish with commonly available mushrooms.

To roast garlic: Preheat the oven to 400°F. Rub unpeeled garlic cloves with cold-pressed olive oil and wrap in foil. Bake until garlic cloves are soft, about 45 minutes. When cool, squeeze roasted garlic cloves from their skins and set aside.

WILD RICE and CREAMED SPINACH
Serves 3–4

1 cup uncooked long-grain brown rice
2 cups Vegetable Stock (page 113) or Campbell's All Natural Stock
1 tablespoon cold-pressed virgin olive oil
½ cup cooked wild rice
½ cup chopped onions
1 cup sliced celery
1 cup sliced mushrooms
2 teaspoons chopped fresh thyme
1 cup torn spinach
½ cup soy milk

pinch sea salt

Cook the long-grain rice in the stock and drain. Heat the oil and sauté both rices with the onions, celery, mushrooms, and thyme until the onions are clear. Combine the spinach, soy milk, and salt in a blender and purée. Pour this over the rice mixture and serve with a fresh salad of your choice.

FRIED RICE with EGG and VEGETABLES
Serves 4

1 cup green peas
½ red bell pepper, sliced into long fine strips
½ cup finely chopped broccoli
½ cup shredded Chinese cabbage
2 tablespoons cold-pressed virgin olive oil
4 scallions/green onions, chopped
1 garlic clove, minced
10 sprigs fresh coriander/cilantro
¼ cup chopped fresh basil leaves
3 tablespoons salt-reduced soy sauce
1 tablespoon chili sauce
1 teaspoon brown sugar
4 cups cold cooked rice
2 free-range eggs, beaten
½ cup mung bean sprouts
1 stalk celery, chopped

Lightly steam the peas, then bell pepper, broccoli, and cabbage for no longer than 5 minutes. In the oil, sauté the scallions/green onions, then add garlic, coriander/cilantro, basil, soy sauce, chili sauce, and sugar and sauté for 3 minutes. Add the precooked rice and beaten eggs and stir in. Lastly add the bean sprouts and celery, stirring constantly until warmed through. Serve with a fresh salad of your choice.

DESSERTS

SENSATIONAL SUMMER FRUIT SALAD

Peel, seed, core and cut into chunks the following fruits: ½ cantaloupe, ½ pineapple, 4 ripe mangoes, 3 bananas, 8 kiwifruit, 4 passion fruit, 1 cup of ripe strawberries, and cover with lemon juice to prevent browning of fruit. Pour over 2 cups freshly squeezed orange juice and serve. You may serve with ice cream made from soya beans or fruit sorbet. You may also serve it with our own Fruit and Nut Cream (page 146). Chill fruit before serving. This is a huge fruit salad and you can use different variations and much smaller amounts if it is just for one or two persons. This is full of vitamin C which is the most important vitamin for liver detoxification, so your liver will love this one.

BANANA MOUSSE
Serves 6

3 frozen ripe bananas, peeled
¼ cup lemon juice
3 cups vanilla soy milk, chilled
2 teaspoons vanilla extract
2 tablespoons (½ oz) granualated gelatin
¼ cup boiling water
3 egg whites (*only use eggs that have been stored under refrigeration*)
1 teaspoon ground nutmeg
LSA, for sprinkling
few sprigs fresh mint

Purée the frozen bananas with the lemon juice. Beat the milk and vanilla extract until thick and creamy, and fold through the banana mixture. Mix gelatin in boiling water then fold through banana mixture. Beat the egg whites until stiff, add the nutmeg and fold into the banana mixture. Pour into individual glass dishes, sprinkle with LSA (page 146) and garnish with sprigs of fresh mint.

BAKED APPLES in SKINS
Serves 6

6 large Granny Smith apples
1 teaspoon ground nutmeg
1 teaspoon ground cinnamon
1 teaspoon chopped crystallized ginger
5 tablespoons seedless raisins
6 dates
1 cup apple juice

Preheat the oven to 350°F. Core the apples, being careful not to pierce the bottom skin. Mix spices, raisins, and dates together and stuff the cavity of each apple with the mixture. Place the apples in the apple juice on a baking tray and bake in the oven for 30 minutes. Pour the juice over the apples prior to serving.

CHERRY and PEACH COMBO
2 lb fresh peaches, sliced (reserve stones and fruit peel)
1 tablespoon honey
2 cups purified water
2 lb large black cherries, stoned

Place peel and stones of peaches into a saucepan with enough water to cover, add the honey and cook for 20 minutes. Push peach mixture through a sieve and set aside.

Add the water, prepared peaches, and cherries to a large saucepan. Simmer slowly until fruits soften, then add the stock set aside from the skins and stones. If desired, add some more honey to simmer with the fruit.

GOURMET'S GREEN FRUIT SALAD
1 cup apple juice
2 cinnamon sticks
grated zest 1 lemon
2 cloves
1 ripe honeydew melon, peeled
6 kiwifruit, peeled
2 Granny Smith apples, peeled
¼ cup lemon juice
1 bunch (about 20) seedless green grapes

Combine apple juice, cinnamon, lemon zest, and cloves in a small saucepan and simmer for 10 minutes. Remove from heat, allow to cool and place in the refrigerator to chill. Meanwhile, slice the melon and kiwi fruit. Thinly slice the apples then toss with the lemon juice. Arrange all the fruit in a large glass bowl. Remove the cinnamon stick and cloves from the juice mixture, then pour the mixture over the fruit. Return the bowl to refrigerator to chill.

WHOLE PEARS in GRAPE JUICE
Serves 6

1 cup dark grape juice
juice and zest 1 orange
½ teaspoon ground nutmeg
¼ teaspoon ground cinnamon
6 cloves
6 medium pears
2 teaspoons arrowroot
sprig of mint, for garnish

Mix the grape juice, orange juice and spices. Peel the pears and leave whole with stems on. Place in a saucepan with the liquid, add the orange zest and simmer gently for 30 minutes, or until pears are tender, basting 2 or 3 times with juice. Mix the arrowroot with a little water and pour into the mixture, stirring until it thickens. Place the pears on a plate and spoon the juice over. Garnish with the mint. May also be served with a fruit sorbet if desired.

MAGIC of MELONS
With a melon scoop, make balls from the following:
1 ripe cantaloupe, 1 ripe honeydew melon, 1 ripe watermelon. Fill the empty watermelon shell with all the different melon balls you have made and chill before serving. This is nice with a fruit sorbet or our own Fruit and Nut Cream (page 146).

NUTTY CREAM

½ cup macadamia nuts
½ cup almonds
½ cup cashews
½ cup sunflower seeds
½ cup sesame seeds
¼ cup cornstarch
1 cup vanilla soy milk
1 teaspoon cold-pressed virgin olive oil
2 teaspoons vanilla extract

Place all nuts and seeds through a grinder or high-powered blender first. Then place all ingredients in a blender and blend at high speed until smooth. Pour into individual dessert glasses and place in the freezer. When mixture is frozen serve as ice cream or by cutting into chunks.

PIKELETS

1 cup self-rising whole wheat flour
2 free-range egg whites, lightly beaten
¾ cup soy milk
1 teaspoon vinegar

Sift the flour into a mixing bowl. Add the egg whites, milk and vinegar. Stir the mixture until the ingredients are well combined, then beat until smooth. Heat a small heavy-based nonstick frying pan, brush with oil, then drop the batter in by tablespoons. Cook until the tops become bubbly, then flip over and cook on the other side until brown. Serve warm or cold with apple sauce or honey and sprinkle with LSA (page 146). You may also serve with Fruit and Nut Cream (page 146) or with a fruit sorbet.

DRIED FRUIT SALAD

12 pitted prunes
12 dried apricots
12 dried figs
½ cup seedless raisins
12 dried peaches or apples
2 cups purified water
4 tablespoons orange juice

4 tablespoons rose water (optional)
½ cup pine kernels (or almonds or pecans or a mixture)

Place the dried fruits in a bowl with the purified water, cover with a dish cloth and leave overnight, then chill in the refrigerator. Drain off excess water. Prior to serving stir in the orange juice, rose water and nuts.

COUSCOUS CAKE with BERRIES
2 cups strawberries, blackberries or blueberries
6 cups apple juice
1 tablespoon vanilla extract
3 cups couscous

Wash the berries gently under cold water and place to dry on a paper towel. Place the apple juice, vanilla, and couscous in a large saucepan and bring to a boil, stirring continuously until the couscous has absorbed all the juices and thickened. Gently fold in the berries while mixture is hot. Rinse a baking pan (approximately 10 x 14 in) and leave undried. Transfer the mixture immediately into the baking pan, place in the refrigerator to chill and set; it takes approximately 3 hours.

RICE CUSTARD
Serves 4

½ cup of rice
2½ cups vanilla soy milk
1 beaten egg
2 tablepoons honey
2 tablepoons grated lemon zest
1 tablepoon grated nutmeg

Preheat the oven to 300°F. Soak the rice in the soy milk for 1 hour in a small ovenproof dish. Mix in the egg, honey, and lemon zest. Sprinkle with the grated nutmeg and bake in the oven for 2½ hours.

TARTY CITRUS SALAD

3 oranges, peeled
1 grapefruit (pink skinned are nicer), peeled
6 mandarin oranges, peeled
1 small pineapple, peeled
1 cup freshly squeezed orange juice
freshly chopped mint leaves, for garnish

Slice the citrus fruit into segments, removing membranes of skin, and place into a bowl. Core the pineapple, dice, and add to the bowl of citrus fruit and mix. Add the orange juice and garnish with the chopped mint.

BANANA CAKE

1⅓ cups ripe bananas, mashed
⅓ cup chopped walnuts
⅓ cup cold-pressed sunflower oil
⅔ cup raisins
¾ cup rolled oat flakes
1 cup wholewheat flour
1 teaspoon vanilla extract
pinch sea salt

Preheat the oven to 375°F. Mix all the ingredients together. The consistency should be soft and moist. Brush the base and sides of a 1 lb loaf tin with oil, then spoon in the cake mixture. Bake for 50 minutes, or until a skewer inserted into the center of the cake comes out clean. Cool for 15 minutes before turning out cake.

SPICY STEWED APPLES

1 cup apple juice
8 Granny Smith apples peeled, cored and sliced
5 tablespoons fresh lemon juice
2 tablespoons honey
1 stick cinnamon
½ teaspoon ground allspice
½ teaspoon ground nutmeg
½ teaspoon vanilla extract
2 heaped tablespoons currants
6 cloves

Place the apple juice and sliced apples in a heavy saucepan with all the other ingredients and bring slowly to a boil, then turn heat down and simmer for 10 minutes until the apples are tender. Remove the cloves prior to serving. These apples are delicious served hot or cold.

BERRY NICE SALAD
Serves 6

4 cups strawberries, hulled
2 cups raspberries
2 cups blackberries
2 cups blueberries
2 cups loganberries
1 cup grape juice

Wash and gently mix all the berries together, add the grape juice, and chill. This is very nice with our Fruit and Nut Cream (page 146)

PANCAKES
Makes approximately 12

2 free-range eggs
2 cups vanilla soy milk
1½ cups whole wheat self-rising flour
2 teaspoons vanilla extract

Beat the eggs with 1 cup of the milk. Sieve in half the flour, then add the rest of the milk and flour alternately. Beat well, removing all lumps and adding the vanilla extract. Let mixture stand for 30 minutes. Brush a crepe pan lightly with cold-pressed virgin olive oil (or use a nonstick pan) then heat the pan. When the pan is hot, pour 1/12 of mixture in. The pancakes are ready to turn over when bubbles appear. Serve with fresh citrus juice and honey, or fresh fruit sprinkled with LSA (page 146), or just enjoy them plain.

PASSIONFRUIT and MELON MOUSSE
Serves 4

1 tablespoon gelatine
½ cup hot water
1 honeydew melon, peeled, seeded, and chopped
¼ cup loosely packed brown raw sugar
½ cup orange juice
pulp of 4 very ripe passionfruit

Place the gelatine into the hot water and stir with a fork until dissolved. Place into a blender with the melon, sugar, and orange juice and blend until smooth and frothy. Transfer to a large serving bowl and fold in the passionfruit pulp. Refrigerate until nearly set, then stir again and return to refrigerator until set.

NUTTY APPLE CRUMBLE
6 Granny Smith apples, peeled, cored, and quartered
1 teaspoon ground allspice
1 tablespoon honey
2 tablespoons water
2 heaped tablespoons rolled oats
1 heaped tablespoon desiccated coconut
1 heaped tablespoon LSA (page 146)
1 heaped tablespoon whole wheat flour
2 teaspoons raw sugar
1 tablespoon soy milk yogurt

Preheat the oven to 350°F. Place the first 4 ingredients into a large saucepan and simmer until the apples are just cooked, then remove and place in an ovenproof dish.

To make the crumble, mix together in a small bowl the remaining ingredients, using just enough of the yogurt to bind the crumble mixture—it should not be too moist.

Sprinkle the crumble mixture evenly over the top of the apples and bake in the oven until the crumble becomes golden, 20–30 minutes.

GOLDEN FRUIT SALAD
Serves 6

1 very ripe papaya, peeled, seeded, and sliced
6 ripe mangoes, peeled, stoned, and sliced
6 peaches, peeled, stoned, and sliced
2 oranges, peeled and segmented
½ cantaloupe, peeled, seeded, and cut into chunks
2 cups freshly squeezed orange juice

Gently mix all the ingredients together, chill and serve. This is nice with our Fruit and Nut Cream (page 146).

CARROT CAKE
1 cup all-purpose flour
¾ teaspoon baking soda
1 teaspoon baking powder
½ teaspoon ground cinnamon
½ teaspoon ground nutmeg
½ teaspoon salt
¾ cup raw sugar
2 large free-range eggs
⅓ cup cold-pressed oil
1 cup grated carrot
13 oz canned crushed pineapple (drain well and discard juice)
¼ cup chopped walnuts

Preheat the oven to 350°F. Thoroughly mix together all the ingredients except the carrots, pineapple, and walnuts. Fold in the carrots, pineapple, and walnuts. Grease and flour a cake tin. Bake in the oven for 35–40 minutes.

Q. What is the difference between Livatone and Livatone Plus?

Livatone

Livatone is a natural liver tonic containing the liver herbs St Mary's Thistle, Globe artichoke and Dandelion, combined with the amino acid taurine, and lecithin. It also contains natural sources of chlorophyll, carotenoids and fibre. It is available in capsule and powder form.

Livatone can be used as a general liver tonic and its benefits include:
An aid to weight loss and fat burning
An aid for those with high blood levels of cholesterol and triglycerides
Reduction of fluid retention and irritable bowel syndrome
As a fibre supplement to reduce constipation and bloating (especially the powder form)
An aid for digestive problems and gall bladder dysfunction

Livatone can be taken by anyone wanting to generally improve the function of their liver, which is a good idea from time to time considering that the liver is the most important organ in the body, and in this day and age is in need of support.

Livatone can be used by people of all ages, including children over 2 years of age. Children under 10 years of age should use the powder dissolved in fruit juice before meals in a dose of 1/4 to 1/3 of a teaspoon twice daily. The dose for adults and children over 10 years of age is one teaspoon of powder twice daily stirred into juice just before meals, or 2 capsules twice daily with water just before meals.

Livatone Plus

Livatone Plus has a very different formula to Livatone, and can be described as a more powerful formula for metabolic problems or dysfunctions of the liver.

Livatone Plus contains the liver herb St Mary's Thistle, combined with sulphur bearing amino acids Taurine, Glycine, Cysteine and Glutamine. Livatone Plus also contains all the important B vitamins and lipotrophic cofactors such as Inositol, Folic acid and Biotin. It contains antioxidants to reduce liver damage and inflammation, such as Green Tea, vitamins C, E and natural betacarotene. It also contains lecithin and broccoli powder to help liver function.

Livatone Plus contains the essential nutrients to support the phase one and two detoxification pathways in the liver.

Livatone Plus is beneficial in the following conditions:

• Poor detoxification capability in the liver. These people often have multiple chemical, drug and food sensitivity. They may have been exposed to liver toxins. These people often have Chronic Fatigue Syndrome.

• Those who work in high-risk occupations which expose them to a high load of potential liver toxins such as petrochemicals, insecticides and solvents. For example painters, hair-dressers, motor mechanics, agricultural workers, foundry workers, plumbers, plant and transport operators, those in the dry cleaning industry, and some process and factory workers. If such workers support the liver with protective supplements they will reduce the risk of liver damage. Safe work practises are also of vital importance to minimise risk of contact exposure.

• Chronic headaches (including migraines) associated with nausea, especially if analgesic use is high.

• Those with skin problems such as inflammatory rashes, itchy skin and brown liver spots.

• Those with unstable blood sugar levels such as hypoglycaemia. These people often have strong sugar cravings and great difficulty sticking to a long-term healthy diet. Unstable blood sugar levels are known as glucose intolerance and this is often a forerunner to Type 11 diabetes. Type 11 diabetes is often associated with obesity and a fatty liver. Livatone Plus helps to stabilise blood sugar levels and makes it much easier to resist sugar cravings and stick to a healthy diet.

• Liver damage from various causes such as:

Viral infections of the liver with hepatitis A, B and C, glandular fever and other chronic viral infections that attack the liver.

Liver inflammation (hepatitis) from toxins, alcohol excess, recreational drugs, analgesic excess and drug induced hepatitis.

Autoimmune liver diseases such as Sclerosing Cholangitis, Primary Biliary Cirrhosis, Chronic Active Hepatitis or connective tissue diseases.

Fatty liver induced by incorrect diet, alcohol or diabetes.

Cirrhosis (scarring) of the liver from multiple causes.

Nodular hyperplasia of the liver

Liver cysts

Gall bladder dysfunction and gallstones.

Livatone Plus is available in capsule and powder form. The regular dosage in adults is half a-teaspoon twice daily stirred into a nice fresh juice just before meals, or 2 capsules twice daily with water just before meals. In children over 2 years of age, Livatone Plus can be used to improve liver function in the above complaints. The dosage for children under 10 years of age is 1/4 to 1/3 of a teaspoon twice daily in fruit juice. Children under 10 find it difficult to swallow capsules and the powder should be used.

Both types of Livatone can be taken long term, as they are all natural products and free of side effects. The occasional person is allergic to psyllium, which is found in Livatone, in which case Livatone Plus should be used. Rarely there may be such a severe allergy to salicylates that the person is unable to take any herbs. Most herbs and plants contain salicylates. If salicylate allergy is severe you will have to avoid all products containing herbs and rely on vitamins and amino acids taken individually.

After taking **Livatone** or **Livatone Plus** for 3 - 4 months you can go onto a maintenance dose which is two capsules daily or half of a teaspoon daily. This can be continued indefinitely if you so desire, particularly if you feel healthier while taking **Livatone** formulas.

When starting any liver tonic it is important to begin with a reduced dose to avoid any strong reactions. These can occur because your liver is eliminating toxins rapidly for the first time in years, or rarely because you may be allergic to one of the ingredients. Beginning doses for both types of **Livatone** are 1/2 a teaspoon daily or one capsule daily. Take this dose for one week and if you continue to feel well you may go up to the regular dose on the second week. The regular dose is two capsules twice daily or one teaspoon twice daily.

CONVERSION TABLE FOR RECIPES AND COOKING.

OUNCES	GRAMS
1	28
2	57
3	85
4	113
5	142
6	170
7	198
8	227
9	255
10	283

For additional amounts select the appropriate conversion above and multiply or add or both. ie. 15 ounces

        = 10 ounces (283 grams)
        + 5 ounces (142 grams)
        = 15 ounces (425 grams)

POUNDS	KILOGRAMS	FAHRENHEIT	CENTIGRADE
1	0.45	200 degrees F	93 degrees C
2	0.91	250 degrees F	121 degrees C
3	1.36	300 degrees F	149 degrees C
4	1.81	350 degrees F	177 degrees C
5	2.27	400 degrees F	204 degrees C
6	2.72	For other temperature conversions,	
7	3.17	use the following formula;	
8	3.63	F to C : subtract 32, then divide by 1.8	
9	4.10	C to F : multiply by 1.8, then add 32	
10	4.54		

KITCHEN MEASURES

Measure	Ounces	Milliliters
One teaspoon =	0.17ounces =	5 milliliters
One tablespoon =	0.5 ounces =	14 milliliters
One cup =	8 ounces =	227 milliliters
One pint =	16 ounces =	454 milliliters
One quart =	32 ounces =	908 milliliters
One gallon =	128 ounces =	3632 milliliters

BIBLIOGRAPHY

Diseases of the Liver and Biliary System. Dr. Sheila Sherlock,
  Blackwell Press
The Physicians Handbook of Clinical Nutrition, Dr. Henry Osiecki,
  Bioconcepts Publishing.
Nutritional Influences on Illness, A sourcebook of clinical research.
  Melvyn R. Werbach. M.D.
The Doctor's Vitamin Encyclopedia.
  Dr. Sheldon Hendler. M.D., PhD.
Milk Thistle
  Floersheim GL et al. Effects of silymarin on liver enzymes and
  blood clotting factors in dogs given a boiled preparation of
  Amanita phalloides. Toxicology and Applied Pharmacology. 46:
  455-462,1978
Valenzuela A. et al. Silymarin protection against hepatic lipid
  peroxidation induced by acute ethanol intoxication in the rat.
  Biochemical Pharmacology 34:2209-2212,1985
Vengerovski A. et al. Liver protective action of silybinene in
  experimental CCL4 poisoning. Farmakologiya Toksikologiya
  50:67-69,1987
Wagner H. Antihepatoxic flavonoids. Progress in Clinical and Biology
  Research. 213:319-331,1986
Meister A. Selective modification of glutathione metabolism. Science
  220:472-477,1983
Osiecki H. Taurine the detoxifying amino acid. Nutrients in profile.
  Bioconcepts Publishing.
Bland J.S. et al. Nutritional up-regulation of hepatic detoxification
  enzymes. The Journal of Applied Nutrition, 1992, 44; No. 3 & 4
Professor Robin Fraser et al, Lipoproteins and the Liver Sieve.
  Hepatology 21:863-874. 1995
  http://www.chmeds.ac.nz/~grogers/liver98.html
Cells of the hepatic sinusoid, Vol. 5.,Kupffer Cell Foundation, P.O
  Box 2215, 2301 CE Leiden. The Netherlands.
Ito T. Recent advances in the study on the fine structure of the
  hepatic sinusoidal wall. A review. Gumna Rep Med Sci
  1973;6:119-163
Wisse E, et al. The liver sieve: considerations concerning the
  structure and function of endothelial fenestrae. Hepatology
  1985;5:683-692
Lieber CS, et al. Role of dietary, adipose and endogenously
  synthesised fatty acids in the pathogenesis of the alcoholic fatty
  liver. J Clin Invest 1966;45:51-62

The Liver and Detoxification

More than ever before in the history of mankind, human beings need to have healthy livers to break down the thousands of toxic chemicals that have insidiously crept into our environment and food chain. The liver is the gateway to the body and in this chemical age its detoxification systems are easily overloaded. Plants are sprayed with toxic chemicals, animals are given potent hormones and antibiotics and food is processed, refined, frozen and over cooked. All this can lead to destruction of delicate vitamins and minerals, which are required for the detoxification pathways in the liver.

The liver is our internal cleanser

Under the microscope the liver appears as a huge filter or sieve, which is designed to remove toxic matter such as dead cells, microorganisms, chemicals, fat globules and sludge from the blood stream as it flows through the liver filter. Inside the liver cells there are sophisticated mechanisms that have evolved over millions of years to break down substances such as drugs, artificial chemicals, pesticides and hormones. Many of the toxic chemicals that enter the body are lipid soluble which means they dissolve only in fatty or oily solutions and not in water. Lipid soluble chemicals have a high affinity for fat tissues and cell membranes, which are made of fatty substances. In these fatty parts of the body toxins may be stored for years being released during times of stress, exercise or fasting. During the release of these toxins, symptoms such as headaches, poor memory, stomach pain, nausea, fatigue dizziness and palpitations may occur.

The liver is designed to convert lipid-soluble chemicals into water-soluble chemicals so that they may then be excreted from the body via watery fluids such as the bile and urine. This conversion is done by a complex system of enzymes that exist inside the liver cells. Basically there are two major detoxification pathways inside the liver cells that utilize these enzymes— they are called the Phase One and Phase Two detoxification pathways.

If these detoxification pathways become overloaded there will be a build up of toxic chemicals in the body. Many of these toxins are fat-soluble and accumulate in fatty body organs such as the brain and endocrine (hormone) glands. This may result in symptoms of brain dysfunction and hormonal imbalances such as infertility, breast pain and lumps, menstrual disturbances, reduced sperm count, adrenal gland exhaustion and early menopause. Many of these chemicals are carcinogenic and have been implicated in the rising incidence of many cancers.

If the liver filter and/or detoxification pathways become inefficient or overloaded, this will cause toxins, dead cells, fat globules and microorganisms to build up to undesirably high levels in the blood stream. This may damage the inner lining of the blood vessel walls leading to cardiovascular disease and also increases the workload of the immune system. The immune system becomes overloaded and irritated causing it to produce excessive inflammatory chemicals, and in some cases auto-antibodies, because it is in a hyper-stimulated state. This may lead to symptoms of immune dysfunction such as allergies, inflammatory diseases, swollen glands, recurrent infections, chronic fatigue syndrome or auto-immune diseases. Some of the more common auto-immune diseases are systemic lupus erythematosus, Hashimotos thyroiditis, vasculitis, scleroderma, rheumatoid arthritis, sclerosing cholangitis and some forms of chronic active hepatitis.

Immune dysfunction is common in today's chemically overloaded environment and is exacerbated by nutritional imbalances inherent in processed and high fat diets. Unfortunately, symptoms of immune dysfunction often get treated by suppressive drugs, and rarely does anyone think about the liver. This seems an incredible oversight because it is obvious that the simplest and most efficient way to cleanse the blood stream and take the load off the immune system is by improving liver function.

Support the Liver's Cleansing Functions

Various nutrients and foods can support the liver's phase one and two detoxification pathways and are of special importance in those with dysfunction of the liver and/or immune system, liver disease or toxic overload.
These are:

Cruciferous vegetables- broccoli, cabbage, brussel sprouts, cauliflower

Antioxidants- Vitamin C, E, natural carotenoids, green tea, milk thistle, dandelion, raw fresh garlic and onions, raw fruits and vegetables and their juices, selenium, zinc

Amino acids- glutamine, glycine, methionine, taurine, cysteine

Vitamin B group- thiamine B1, riboflavine B2, nicotinamide B3, pantothenate B5, pyridoxine B6, cyanocobalamin B12, folic acid, biotin, inositol

<u>Essential fatty acids</u>- primrose oil, flaxseed (linseed) oil or ground seeds, fresh wheatgerm and lecithin, avocados, cold pressed olive oil, raw fresh seeds and nuts, oily fish, legumes (beans, peas and lentils). Legumes are also a good source of the amino acid arginine, which helps the liver to detoxify ammonia.

Research is currently going on to develop formulas of new Livatone products which enhance and support the liver's detoxification pathways and also help those with liver disease. To stay current with these ongoing developments you may look us up on the world wide web at http://www.whas.com.au or http://www.liverdoctor.com
Or in the U.S.A. call 1-888-782-7014 or 1-888-75LIVER
Or elsewhere call Australia 61-246-531445 or Fax 61-246-531144

INTERNATIONAL CONTACT DETAILS

U.S.A.
S.C.B. International
PO Box 5070 Glendale AZ
85312 - 5070
Phone: 1-888-75LIVER or 6233343232
Web site: http://www.liverdoctor.com
Email: usahelp@qwest.net
G.K. Products
10088 N.W. 3rd Place, Coral Springs, FLA 33071
Phone: 1-888-752-4286

AUSTRALIA
Health Advisory Service
P.O. Box 54, Cobbitty, NSW, 2570
Phone: 61-246-531445   Fax: 61-246-531144
Email-cabot@ozemail.com.au
Web site-http://www.whas.com.au or http://www.liverdoctor.com

NEW ZEALAND
Thompsons Nutrition
Suppliers of Livatone and Selenomune
25 Constellation Dve, Mairangi Bay, Auckland 10, N.Z.
Phone: 64-94785921, Fax: 64-94785991
Penguin Books
Phone: 64-94154700, Fax: 64-94154701

UNITED KINGDOM
Deep Books, Unit 13, Cannon Wharf Business Centre
35 Evelyn St. London SE85 RT
Phone: 44-1712322747 or freecall 0845-6010245, or 44-1718379911
Fax: 44-1712370067
Holistic Medical Clinic – "The Grove"
182-184 Kensington Church St. W8 4DP
Phone: 44-171-2212266, Fax 44-171-2432112
British Liver Trust
Phone: 44-1473276326 or 44-1473276328
Fax: 44-1473276327

BOOST YOUR ENERGY!

Selenomune *Designer Energy Powder* is packed with immune boosting nutrients to help the energy factories inside your cells to produce more energy.

Selenomune contains:
Minerals - selenium, zinc, manganese, chromium, boron, molybdenum, calcium, magnesium
Anti-oxidants - Vitamins C and E and carotenoids.
Synergistic nutrients - malic acid, B group vitamins, amino acids, biotin, folic acid, chlorophyll, kelp in a special designer yeast powder. This is a healthy yeast for the gut, and is a well absorbed form of trace minerals.
Take one or two teaspoons daily, stirred into fresh juices, just before eating meals.
Selenomune is available in **New Zealand** from Thompsons Nutrition, 25 Constellation Dve, Malrangi Bay, Auckland 10, phone 64-9-4785921 or in the **United States of America** from SCB Int. Po Box 5070 Glendale AZ 85312 - 5070, Phone 623-334-3232 or 1-888-75LIVER.

SUPERFOOD FOR MENOPAUSE
FEMMEPHASE

Femmephase contains minerals, anti-oxidants, herbs and foods to help you pass through the years before, during, and after menopause. It contains four different types of **calcium** to strengthen the bones and nails. It is high in **trace minerals** and is good for those with hair loss, as it helps to strengthen hair. It is also helpful for those with a sluggish metabolism.
Femmephase contains **natural plant hormones**.
Femmephase contains a large range of herbs such as licorice, black cohosh, sage, wild yam and dong qual which have been used successfully for female complaints for centuries. These herbs are a source of **NATURAL PLANT ESTROGENS**.

Femmephase is available in the U.S.A. from SCB International by calling 1-888-75LIVER.

SHOPPING/GROCERY LIST FOR LIVER LOVERS

If possible try to buy produce that is organically grown and raised and is fresh and free of chemical preservatives. This is not always possible so do the best you can. Your local health food store will be a good source of information in these matters.

Liver friendly foods
- Raw and dried fruits.
- Raw vegetables. Vegetables that are highly liver cleansing because of their high sulfur content are cruciferous vegetables (broccoli, brussel sprouts, cabbage, cauliflower) and garlic and onions. Fruits and vegetables with deep bright pigments such as orange, yellow, red and green colors are very cleansing (eg. Carrots, pumpkin, citrus fruits, red cabbage, red and green peppers). Mushrooms, potatoes, yams, avocado, olives, sea weeds,
- Raw nuts such as brazil, almonds, cashews and walnuts.
- Raw seeds such as flaxseed (linseeds), sunflower, sesame, pumpkin seeds.
- Legumes, which consist of beans, lentils and peas. These can be raw or sprouted.
- Sprouts–alfalfa, mung bean, wheat grass, barley grass are a good source of chlorophyll which is liver cleansing.
- Grains such as wheat, buckwheat, rye, barley, oats, quinoa, rice.
- Breads–- whole-grain, multi-grain, stone ground, pita, sourdough. Biscuits–- crisp breads and crackers made from whole-grains that are free of hydrogenated vegetable oils and fat. May be salt free or lightly salted. Avoid sweet biscuits. Pastas made from whole-grains.
- Chicken, preferably free range and don't forget to remove the skin!
- Eggs, preferably free range.
- Seafoods such as tuna, salmon, sardines, mackerel (oily fish), fresh fish fillets, shellfish. Canned fish is healthy. Avoid eating seafood raw, smoked or deep-fried.
- Spreads for breads/biscuits– hummus, tahini, nut spreads such as brazil, almond, cashew, honey, natural fruit jams, fresh avocado.
- Cold pressed virgin vegetable and seed oils eg. olive, flaxseed, safflower, sunflower, canola, grapeseed, etc.
- Beverages: soy milk, almond milk, oat milk, rice milk, water (filtered, distilled or purified), bottled or canned fruit and vegetable juices with no added sugar, tea (regular, green or herbal). Tea tastes quite nice with soy milk.
- Spices if desired–- chili, ginger, coriander, curry, cayenne, tumeric, basil, rosemary, fennel and others if they are natural.

Kitchen utensils needed to follow liver cleansing diet
Juice extracting machine for making fresh raw juices.
(Good juice combinations are carrot, celery, beets and apple).
Orange juice squeezer.
Coffee grinder or food processor for grinding seeds and nuts.
Blender for making smoothies and soups.
Water filter or purifier.
Shop wisely with liver consciousness. Love your liver and live longer!